MYELOFIBROSIS

HEMATOLOGY

Series Editor

Kenneth M. Brinkhous, M.D.
Department of Pathology
University of North Carolina
School of Medicine
Chapel Hill, North Carolina

Volume 1 Prostaglandins and Leukotrienes: Blood and Vascular Cell Function, *Jonathan M. Gerrard*

Volume 2 Hematopoietic Stem Cells, *edited by David W. Golde and Fumimaro Takaku*

Volume 3 Bone Marrow Transplantation: Biological Mechanisms and Clinical Practice, *edited by Dirk W. van Bekkum and Bob Löwenberg*

Volume 4 Myelofibrosis: Pathophysiology and Clinical Management, *edited by S. M. Lewis*

Other Volumes in Preparation

MYELOFIBROSIS

Pathophysiology and Clinical Management

edited by
S. M. LEWIS
Department of Haematology
Royal Postgraduate Medical School
University of London
London, England

MARCEL DEKKER, INC. New York • Basel

Library of Congress Cataloging in Publication Data

Main entry under title:

Myelofibrosis : pathophysiology and clinical management.

(Hematology ; v. 4)
Based on a symposium held at the Annual General Meeting of the British Society for Haematology in Leeds in Apr. 1983.
Includes index.
1. Myelofibrosis--Congresses. I. Lewis, S. M. (Shirley Mitchell) II. British Society for haematology. General Meeting (1983 : Leeds, West Yorkshire) III. Series: Hematology (New York, N.Y.) ; v. 4. [DNLM: 1. Myelofibrosis--physiopathology--congresses. W1 HE873 v.4 / WH 380 M9967 1983]
RC645.76.M95 1985 616.4'1 85-10198
ISBN 0-8247-7411-6

MARCEL DEKKER, INC.
270 Madison Avenue, New York, New York 10016

Current printing (last digit):
10 9 8 7 6 5 4 3 2 1

PRINTED IN THE UNITED STATES OF AMERICA

Introduction to the Series

Hematology as a field has followed a pattern for most of this century of major scientific discoveries, improved understanding of disease, and rapid applications of new knowledge in the clinic. Advances continue at an accelerating pace, so that all but the most zealous have difficulty in keeping up with the literature in even a limited area of specialized interest. As the explosive development of knowledge continues apace, it is a continuing challenge to keep abreast of significant new developments as they impact on clinical and laboratory hematology. The Hematology series is designed to help in this respect, by providing up-to-date and expert presentations of important subject areas in our field. It is hoped that these works, both individually and collectively, will become important volumes to update one's information and for reference for the clinician, investigator, teacher, and student, and in this manner contribute to the advancement of hematology.

The present volume deals with a long-recognized and often puzzling disorder, myelofibrosis. It has been over a century since this condition was separated from the leukemias by Heuck. The acute form of the disease was described in 1963 by the editor of this volume, Dr. S. M. Lewis. Known by many names, it is now usually referred to as primary or idiopathic myelofibrosis with myeloid metaplasia or less commonly today, agnogenic myeloid metaplasia. The many outstanding experts who have contributed to this volume have provided a lucid and "state of the art" presentation of the various features and basic concepts of the disease. The chapters on pathology and pathophysiology, clinical manifestations, and management well reflect the current state of knowledge of this condition. Of special interest are the basic findings in myelofibrosis related to topics such as the presence of colony-stimulating hematopoietic growth factors, the varied cytogenetic findings distinct from chronic myelogenous leukemia (CML), and the possible relation of fibrous tissue proliferation to the release of platelet-derived growth factor (PDGF) from megakaryocytes and platelets. From these data comes the distinct impression that the disease, whether in either its acute or chronic form, is basically one of clonal proliferation, often with a prominent megakaryocytic component pathologically, with the prominent fibrosis and osteosclerosis being secondary phenomena. The syndrome of myelofibrosis and osteosclerosis, extramedullary hematopoiesis and splenomegaly, and a leukoerythroblastic blood picture, repeatedly observed in myelofibrosis, is also observed in many other conditions, including other myeloproliferative disorders, nonhematologic malignancies, infections, and irradiation injury. The comparisons of these conditions with myelofibrosis are especially valuable.

Kenneth M. Brinkhous, M.D.
Series Editor

Preface

Primary chronic myelofibrosis has been, to some extent, the Cinderella of the myeloproliferative disorders. Thus, it has not attracted the research and clinical endeavors that have been devoted to the leukemias; there have been few serious therapeutic trials despite its poor prognosis and unsatisfactory response to any of the treatments which have been used. It is a confusing disease, as is well demonstrated by the multiplicity of names by which it has been identified in the literature. Relatively easy to diagnose morphologically, it is much more difficult to assign a pathogenesis and to be sure that there is a difference between "primary myelofibrosis" and marrow fibrosis due to a reactive process.

However, increasing attention is now being given to this condition first recognized over 100 years ago. Experimental studies are beginning to define the true nature of marrow fibrosis and the collagen deposition, which is the invariable pathological lesion. Clinical and morphological observations together with cell culture studies are establishing the essential features that constitute the clinical syndrome and are identifying the role of hematopoietic progenitor cells, especially megakaryopoiesis, in the pathogenesis of myelofibrosis and the occurrence of acute (malignant) myelofibrosis.

This aroused interest encouraged the British Society for Haematology to have a symposium on the subject at the Annual General Meeting of the Society in Leeds in April 1983. That symposium has been the basis for this monograph. The speakers at the symposium were invited to contribute chapters based on their oral presentations and the contents were expanded with additional contributions to provide a comprehensive survey of various aspects of the subject taking into account the viewpoint of the clinician, morphologist, electronmicroscopist, experimental hematologist, cytogeneticist, and nuclear medicine physician.

I was privileged to be chairman of the British Society for Haematology symposium and it was a pleasure to accept the subsequent invitation to edit this book as one in the Marcel Dekker Hematology Series.

In a multiauthored book on a single theme, it is inevitable that there will be a certain amount of repetition between chapters unless the editor applies a rigid discipline. There are, however, important advantages in not applying that discipline too rigidly. First of all it is desirable that each chapter should be complete in its own right and, secondly, if duplication demonstrates areas of disagreement between authors, the reader will appreciate that there are still areas of uncertainty to be explored and that the subject is not yet definite and ready for a didactic textbook. Relevant cross-referencing has been made.

The editor is grateful to all contributors who have, as conscientiously as possible, kept to the time schedule and by their cooperation and helpfulness have made the task of editing easy and trauma free.

S. M. Lewis

Contributors

Reiner Bartl, M.D. Division of Internal Medicine, City Centre Hospital, University of Munich, Munich, West Germany

Stuart A. Bentley, M.D. Department of Pathology, University of North Carolina, Chapel Hill, North Carolina

G. J. den Ottolander, M.D. Department of Haematology, Leiden University Medical Center, Leiden, The Netherlands

Augustin Ferrant, M.D. Departments of Haematology and Nuclear Medicine, University of Louvain Medical School, Brussels, Belgium

Bertha Frisch, M.D. Institute of Haematology, Ichilov Hospital, Tel Aviv Medical Centre, Tel Aviv, Israel

Colin G. Geary, M.A.M.B.,F.R.C.P.,F.R.C.Path. University Department of Haematology, The Royal Infirmary, Manchester, England

John M. Goldman, D.M. Medical Research Council, Leukaemia Unit, Royal Postgraduate Medical School, Hammersmith Hospital, London, England

Jill A. Hibbin, D.Phil. Medical Research Council, Leukaemia Unit, Royal Postgraduate Medical School, Hammersmith Hospital, London, England

M. Imbert, M.D. Service Central d'Hématologie-Immunologie, Hôpital Henri Mondor, Creteil, France

Sylvia D. Lawler, M.D. Section of Human Genetics, Institute of Cancer Research and Department of Cytogenetics, Royal Marsden Hospital, London, England

S. M. Lewis, M.D.,F.R.C.Path. Department of Haematology, Royal Postgraduate Medical School, University of London, London, England

F. Sigaux, M.D.,F.R.C.Path. Service Central d'Hématologie-Immunologie, Hopital Henri Mondor, Creteil, France

Murray N. Silverstein, M.D. Division of Hematology, Mayo Medical School, Rochester, Minnesota

C. Sultan, M.D. Service Central d'Hématologie-Immunologie, Hôpital Henri Mondor, Creteil, France

G. John Swansbury, B.Sc. Department of Cytogenetics, Royal Marsden Hospital, London, England

Contents

MYELOFIBROSIS

1

Myelofibrosis: Historical Perspective

S. M. LEWIS
Royal Postgraduate Medical School, University of London, London, England

TERMINOLOGY

There have been an extraordinary number of synonyms used in the literature to describe the condition that is the subject to be treated in this monograph (1). This number reflects the complexity of the clinical presentation of myelofibrosis, and it reflects, too, the considerable argument with regard to its pathogenesis and speculation whether it is a single disease or a syndrome, or one of a group of interrelated conditions. Thus, over the years, in various case reports and reviews, the condition has been referred to as: agnogenic myeloid metaplasia, aleukemic myelosis, chronic erythroblastosis, chronic nonleukemic myelosis, chronic splenomegaly with anemia and myeloid reaction in the blood, generalized osteosclerosis, hematopoietic splenomegaly with marrow sclerosis, leukoerythroblastic anemia with diffuse osteosclerosis, megakaryocytic myelosis with osteosclerosis, megakaryocytic splenomegaly, myelofibrosis, myelogenous pseudoleukemia, myeloid megakaryoctic hepatosplenomegaly, myeloid splenic anemia, myelosclerosis, osteomyelosclerosis, osteosclerotic anemia, osteosclerotic leukemia, splenomegalic myelophthisis, and splenomegaly with marrow sclerosis.

In view of the characteristic chronic course of this condition and, as will be described below, the fact that the constant features are bone marrow fibrosis, which is not necessarily accompanied by sclerosis, and extramedullary hematopoiesis, perhaps the most apt name for this condition is "chronic myelofibrotic myeloid metaplasia." However, in recent years the terms "chronic myelofibrosis" and "primary myelofibrosis" have come into favor. The former is descriptive without implying what pathogenetic mechanism might be responsible, although it does not take account of the acute form of the disorder (see later). The latter, on the other hand, does not take into account the possibility that the myelofibrosis may be, invariably, a secondary phenomenon. In this chapter, the term "primary myelofibrosis" (PMF) will be used.

The first record of a case that almost certainly was one of PMF appears to have been that reported by G. H. Heuck (2) in 1879 in *Virchow's Archives* in a paper entitled "Zeuei Fälle vor Leukämie mit eigenthümlichen Blut-resp. Knockenmarksbefund." The patient was a 24-year-old man who had been suffering from severe fatigue for a year. On examination he was found to have a marked hepatosplenomegaly, severe anemia, and leukocytosis with several immature cells in the blood. Two years later he died of pleurisy. Postmortem examination revealed a large spleen and liver; in the diaphyses of the long bones, the cortex was thick, and the medullary cavity was narrow and filled with spongy tissue. In the intratrabecular spaces there was bone marrow that resembled connective tissue. All bones appeared to have been similarly affected and there was pronounced hematopoiesis in the spleen and liver. The pathology was judged to be osteosclerosis and Heuck concluded that it was a chance finding which he believed was unrelated to the presumed leukemia.

Other cases were then recognized as conforming to same picture, and 20 years later in 1899, it was clearly distinguished from leukemia by P. Baumgarten (3) who, in a paper entitled "Myelogene Pseudoleukämie mit Ausgang in allgemeine Osteosclerose," gave a full clinical and histological description of a patient, a 58-year-old man, with the features of PMF.

Over the years, thereafter, there was an increasing number of case reports and the clinical and hematological syndrome began to be recognized, and especially the presence of marrow fibrosis. By the 1950s, coincident with advances in histological staining procedures, and their use in conjunction with bone marrow biopsies, increasing attention was paid to the fibrosis. The designation "myelofibrosis" began to be established to describe the syndrome, to highlight the fact that it was now generally agreed that it was the replacement of bone marrow by connective tissue that was the pathognomonic lesion, and that this might not always be accompanied by sclerosis. This understanding was advanced by major contributions in studies of the bone marrow by various authors (4-9).

HISTOLOGY

The histological features were reviewed and defined by Andreason (8), Lennert (9), and others who have, in general, agreed in their descriptions of what characterizes the pathological features of the bone marrow in PMF. These can be divided into nonfibrotic and fibrotic. In the former, there are qualitative and quantitative changes in all types of cells, but especially in myelopoiesis, erythropoiesis, megakaryocytes, and reticulum cells. These changes are sometimes minimal, but in other cases they may be marked. At first there is hyperplasia of all cells, usually with a normal relative distribution. At a later stage, there is a decreasing number of hematopoietic cells and reticulum cells with an increased fat content, and this is accompanied by the beginning of fibroblast proliferation. Subsequently, the fibrotic features begin to predominate. Calcification of the fibrous ground substance occurs, large and atypical osteocytes appear, and the increasing fibrosis is paralleled by depletion of hematopoietic cells. The striking presence of megakaryocytes at this late stage was noted in some early reviews, and the abnormal morphology was commented on, giving rise to speculation that this might be the essence of the disease by Favre et al. (10) who named the disease "la myelose aleucemique megacaryocytaire," and by Hittmair (11), who referred to it as "megacaryocytenleukämie und Osteomyelosklerose."

The relatively simple histological technique by means of which reticulin may be demonstrated and also its obviously constant increase in PMF encouraged extensive studies of this aspect of the disease (1, 6, 12-16). Early workers identified reticulin as a precursor of collagen, and recognized its presence in a section as evidence of the earliest phase of connective tissue formation. From earlier histological studies, it was appreciated that the connective tissue framework of normal bone marrow consists of a network of fine reticulin fibers. It was then recognized that an increase in reticulin occurred in several diseases other than PMF and it was suggested that there were two distinct patterns: (a) a quantitative increase of fine branching fibers laid out in an essentially normal pattern and (b) an abnormal design consisting of a coarse mesh of argyrophilic fibers that are thicker than normal and that follow a wavy course, aggregating into bundles of parallel fibers with the morphology of collagen (17). The former pattern was found in association with hypercellularity per se, whereas the latter pattern was reputed to occur predominantly in PMF and also, to some extent, in polycythemia vera, chronic myeloid leukemia, and multiple myeloma.

These disease-linked differences in the reticulin pattern are sometimes tenuous and do not always stand up to close scrutiny; there was need for a more refined method of analysis of the type of material and for determining the relationship of "reticulin" to collagen. Immunohistochemical studies of normal human bone marrow have shown that collagen types I and III are normally distributed within the hematopoietic compartment of bone marrow whereas type IV collagen is localized to the endothelial lining of sinusoids and the blood vessels (18). The so-called reticulin staining by silver impregnation appears not to be a specific connective tissue protein stain as originally thought, but it stains a glycoprotein or proteoglycan matrix that is associated with fine connective tissue fibers (19). This view is not entirely supported by

Table 1 Histological Course of Primary Chronic Myelofibrosis

1. Cellular phase
   a. Diffusely hyperplastic; normal maturation of erythropoiesis and granulopoiesis
   b. Megakaryocytes may predominante; some immature forms
   c. Reticulin ± increase
2. Fibrotic phase
   a. Megakaryocytes still predominant; decreasing numbers of other hemopoietic cells
   b. Altered sinus architecture
   c. Reticulin ++
   d. Collagen +
3. Sclerotic phase
   a. Grossly disturbed architecture
   b. Markedly reduced hematopoiesis
   c. Megakaryocyte/megakaryoblast clusters
   d. Fibroblasts +++
   e. Reticulin +++
   f. Collagen +++
4. Osteosclerotic phase
   a. Fibroblasts +++
   b. Collagen +++
   c. Osteocyte proliferation with bone formation

Charron et al. (20) on the basis of a parallel biochemical and histological analysis of the bone marrow that they carried out. They demonstrated that in early myelofibrosis there is an increase in neutral soluble collagen; as the disease progresses, the hydroxyproline increases and the collagen changes to a polymeric form that is more stable, insoluble, and cross-linked. Hydroxyproline reflects proteoglycan and glycoprotein content of tissues known to be associated with collagen in the intercellular matrix (21) and the correlation demonstrated by Charron et al. (20) (in both normal controls and myelofibrosis) suggests that reticulin staining does depend on the amount of collagen present. Other studies have indicated that reticulin is formed by collagen fibers (collagen III) intimately associated with other connective tissue components such as fibronectin. Charron's conclusion was that in early PMF there is type III (soluble) collagen and that this is replaced by type I collagen in later stages. As this latter form is cross-linked and insoluble, it is irreversible, and thus influences the progression of the disease. It is this type that occurs in osteosclerosis (22–23). The histological course of PMF is summarized in Table 1.

THE CLINICAL SYNDROME

The clinical syndrome has been described in a number of published papers. Wyatt and Somers (5) reported on a series of 30 cases and noted previously published records of some 129 cases. Subsequent reviews have included those of Korst et al. (24), Linman and Bethell (25), Bouroncle and Doan (26), Ward and Block (27), Takácsi-Nagy and Graf (28), and most recently Varki et al. (29). All of these reports draw attention to the fact that whereas diagnosis requires demonstration of the presence of fibrosis in a bone marrow biopsy, this may not always be simple because of the patchy nature of the fibrosis, at least in the early stages. A leukoerythroblastic blood picture and "tear-drop" poikilocytic-shaped erythrocytes are characteristic features, but they are not always present. There is almost always splenomegaly, often marked, by the time the patient has reason to consult a physician, and even in the few patients who present without splenomegaly, this develops in the course of time. Hepatomegaly also occurs in a high proportion of patients (see Table 2).

The triad of leukoerythroblastic anemia, poikilocytosis, and splenomegaly suggests the occurrence of extramedullary erythropoiesis. The spleen is the predominant site in which this occurs. The spleen plays an important multifactorial role in PMF, and investigation of splenic function by means of radionuclides has become important for assessing and measuring (a) splenic red cell pooling, (b) splenic red cell sequestration and destruction, (c) the effect of

Table 2 Clinical and Hematological Features in Primary Chronic Myelofibrosis at Time of Diagnosis, in Some Published Series

<table>
<tr><th></th><th>Andreason (7)</th><th>Bouroncle and Doan (26)</th><th>Korst et al. (24)</th><th>Linman and Bethel (25)</th></tr>
<tr><td>Number of Cases</td><td>56</td><td>100</td><td>23</td><td>53</td></tr>
<tr><td>Splenomegaly (%)</td><td></td><td></td><td></td><td></td></tr>
<tr><td>0</td><td>23</td><td>6</td><td>0</td><td>2</td></tr>
<tr><td>+</td><td>14</td><td>24</td><td>13</td><td>5</td></tr>
<tr><td>++</td><td>24</td><td>21</td><td>13</td><td>40</td></tr>
<tr><td>+++</td><td>39</td><td>49</td><td>74</td><td>53</td></tr>
<tr><td>Hepatomegaly (%)</td><td></td><td></td><td></td><td></td></tr>
<tr><td>0</td><td>60</td><td>29</td><td>0</td><td>10</td></tr>
<tr><td>+</td><td>20</td><td>56</td><td>30</td><td rowspan="2">77</td></tr>
<tr><td>++</td><td>20</td><td>12</td><td>52</td></tr>
<tr><td>+++</td><td>0</td><td>3</td><td>18</td><td>13</td></tr>
<tr><td>Lymph nodes palpable (%)</td><td>25</td><td>12</td><td>25</td><td>5</td></tr>
<tr><td>Leukoerythroblastic anemia (%)</td><td>91</td><td>"Majority of cases"</td><td>96</td><td>75</td></tr>
<tr><td>Tear-drop poikilocytes (%)</td><td>73</td><td>"Characteristic"</td><td>78</td><td>100</td></tr>
</table>

Grades of splenomegaly and hepatosplenomegaly as recorded in the publications: 0 = not palpable; + = "slight"; palpable < 5 cm below costal margin; ++ = "moderate"; palpable 5–10 cm; +++ = "marked"; palpable > 10 cm and including cases reported as "massive enlargements."

hypersplenism on platelet kinetics and the peripheral platelet count, (d) the presence of residual marrow function and the degree of extramedullary erythropoiesis, and (e) whether the erythropoiesis is effective or ineffective (30–32). Furthermore, in PMF there is frequently an expanded plasma volume so that direct measurement of red cell volume is necessary to distinguish between true anemia and hypervolemic (pseudo) anemia.

An association of extramedullary hematopoiesis with PMF was noted in several of the reviews referred to above. It would appear to be an essential diagnostic feature.

Extramedullary erythropoiesis may occur in a wide variety of conditions as a consequence of two different mechanisms. It is common in children in association with severe chronic anemia, for whatever cause, but it is less common in adults under similar circumstances. This is, presumably, a compensatory phenomenon. The second mechanism is a proliferative process that is not directly related to the degree of anemia. Myeloproliferative disorders, tuberculosis, carcinomatosis, and benzene toxicity are all in this category and are all associated with marrow fibrosis. It should, however, be remarked that marrow fibrosis, per se, does not necessarily or invariably induce extramedullary hematopoiesis, whereas it is a constant feature in PMF, which for this reason has been termed agnogenic myeloid metaplasia (33).

VARIANTS OF MYELOFIBROSIS

In 1939, Vaughan and Harrison (12) studied the histology of a series of patients with leukoerythroblastic anemia; they suggested that "polythaemia, megakaryocytic leukaemia and myelosclerosis" were a closely related group of diseases. Just how close was defined by Dameshek (34) in 1951 in his classic editorial in *Blood* in which he proposed the term "myeloproliferative disorders" and speculated on a common myelostimulatory factor linking "agnogenic myeloid metaplasia of spleen" to chronic granulocytic leukemia, polycythemia vera, erythroleukemia, and megakaryocytic leukemia. He remarked on the difficulty of making clear-cut division because "so many transition forms exist." Various published papers, before and after, have drawn attention to the transformation of one condition to another, and especially of polycythemia vera to leukemia or PMF (27, 35–41) (Table 3). Pettit et al. (42) reported the course in a remarkable patient, a 67-year-old woman who had polycythemia vera for 21 years. This transformed to myelofibrosis with massive splenomegaly, but following treatment with splenic irradiation and alkylating agents her spleen became smaller, although it was still significantly enlarged. She again became polycythemic; the bone marrow showed hyperplastic erythropoiesis and granulopoiesis without fibrosis. Extramedullary erythropoiesis, which had been present earlier, was no longer demonstrable by ^{52}Fe ferrokinetic studies. Subsequently (43), a group of 11 patients were seen with some clinical features of both polycythemia vera and PMF at the same time. They had elevated red cell volume, moderate to marked splenomegaly, leukoerythroblastic blood picture, tear-drop poikilocytes, bone marrow with hypercellular hematopoiesis, but also with markedly increased reticulin and extramedullary erythropoiesis. This transitional

Table 3 Transformation of Polycythemia Vera

	Total number of patients	Leukemia	(%)	PMF	(%)
RPMS, London					
ref. 36 (1966)	169	4	2.4	12	7.1
data updated (1978)	200	8	4	18	9
Inst. Gustave-Roussy, Villejuif					
ref. 37 (1968)	296	33	11	16	5.4
PV Study Group					
ref. 41 (1981)	431	26	6	5	1.2
Total[a]	927	67	7.2	39	4.2

[a]RPMS 1978 data include the earlier (1966) data.

syndrome was not necessarily the beginning of transformation into classic PMF because most of the patients remained in a steady state with unchanging features for at least several years.

One of the main problems in considering the question of transformation within the myeloproliferative disorders is that of the definition of the clinical entities. Taking Pettit's cases into account, it seems appropriate to refer to those cases in which there is a unique relationship between their polycythemia vera features and PMF features as "transitional myeloproliferative disorder." It is not known how uncommon such cases are, but a further study of them might advance our understanding of the natural history of the myeloproliferative disorders.

Another facet of this complex subject relates to so-called "malignant" or acute myelofibrosis. Classically, PMF is a chronic disorder, progressive, but usually of several years duration before the (usually) inevitable fatal outcome. In 1963, Lewis and Szur (44) described five cases that presented with an acute rapidly progressive illness and showed the histological features of PMF, but with a blood picture suggestive of acute leukemia with anemia, thrombocytopenia, and leucopenia with a small proportion of blasts. Neither spleen nor liver was palpable. They called this condition "malignant myelofibrosis." They noted and illustrated the prominence of "giant cells similar to megakaryocytes" in the marrow. There were subsequent reports of similar cases (45-50). Efrati et al. (51) described a patient with myelofibrosis terminating in acute micromegakaryoblastic leukemia. In the same year, Den Ottolander et al. (52) investigated three patients with presenting features similar to malignant myelofibrosis and who were subsequently shown, by cytochemistry and electron microscopy, to have megakaryoblastic leukemia. They concluded that acute or malignant myelofibrosis is a secondary phenomenon, the basic event being megakaryoblastic proliferation. This was supported by Bain et al. (53) who also demonstrated megakaryoblast proliferation in four cases of acute myelofibrosis. Whether this is the essential lesion in all such cases is not clear. It is known that platelets secrete a factor (platelet-derived growth factor, PDGF) which stimulates collagen synthesis by mesenchymal cells (23, 54-56), but other factors are also capable of inducing fibrosis, so that only where megakaryoblasts have been identified should this be claimed as the pathogenetic factor.

Categorization within the myeloproliferative spectrum is not yet completely defined. Bone marrow culture studies are beginning to throw some light on the relationship of fibroblast proliferation, marrow fibrosis, and proliferation of normal and abnormal hematopoietic progenitor cells. These studies provide further evidence that the fibrosis is reactive and that the primary cause is a clonal disorder in one or the other hematopoietic stem cell (57).

IMMUNE COMPLEXES

There has been a small interest in immune complexes in relation to myelofibrosis. Lewis and Pegrum (58) found intracellular immune complexes in the peripheral leukocytes in all of 14 patients with PMF, in contrast to negative findings in other myeloproliferative disorders. They postulated that this occurs on an autoimmune basis. These findings were confirmed by Caligaris Cappio et al. (59) who found immunoglobulin G (IgG) as the main immunoglobulin class in the composition of complexes; they suggested a mechanism whereby the immune complexes interact with platelets causing discharge of PDGF with ensuing mesenchymal cell activation and fibrosis.

A range of immune disorders (antinuclear and antismooth muscle autoantibodies, rheumatoid factor, increased serum immunoglobulin levels, positive direct Coombs test, anti-I autoantibody) were found in a group of 67 patients with myelofibrosis by Rondeau et al. (60) who observed that the more frequent and numerous these abnormalities, the more severe is the myelofibrosis, suggesting a lymphoid cell involvement and supporting the concept of immune mechanisms in the pathogenesis of myelofibrosis.

CONCLUSION

At first myelofibrosis was considered to be merely an unusual histological phenomenon of anecdotal interest alone. Even later, PMF was viewed as a fairly rare clinical syndrome and it elicited little interest even though its failure to respond to various therapeutic approaches should have been a much greater stimulus to more hematologists to study this problem. In recent years, however, it has come to be seen as an important topic in experimental hematology, to play an important part in the pathophysiology of hematopoietic cells, and to have a key linking role in the myeloproliferative disorders. Thus, increasingly, attention is being paid to it. This introduction is intended to provide an historical background to the subject. In the chapters that follow, the authors expand on the different aspects that have been touched on superficially here and they provide reviews of present-day concepts of diagnosis, clinical hematological and histopathological features, and treatment. They also describe recent experimental work by means of which questions relating to pathogenesis and other problems are being elucidated.

REFERENCES

1. Erf, L. A., and Herbut, P. A. (1944). Primary and secondary myelofibrosis. *Ann. Int. Med. 21*: 863–889.
2. Heuck, G. (1879). Zwei Fälle von Leukämie mit eigenthümlichen Blut-resp. Knochenmarksbefund. *Virch. Arch. Path. Anat. 78*: 475–496.
3. Baumgarten, P. (1899). Myelogene Pseudoleukämie mit Ausgang in allgemeine Osteosklerose. Arbeit aus der pathologie Institut, *Tübingen 2*: 499–528.
4. Moeschlin, S. (1949). Leucémes myéloides et pseudo-leucémies: Ostéocléroses et myélofibroses. Leur diagnostic différentiel par la ponction de la rate. *Rev. Méd. Suisse Rom. 69*: 633–643.
5. Wyatt, J. P., and Somers, S. C. (1950). Chronic marrow failure, myelosclerosis and extramedullary hematopoiesis. *Blood 5*: 329–347.
6. Peace, R. J. (1953). Myelosclerosis, extramedullary myelopoiesis and leucoerythroblastosis. *Am. J. Pathol. 29*: 1029–1057.
7. Black-Schaffer, B., and Stoddard, L. D. (1953). Panmyelosis and chronic granulocytic leukemia. *Am. J. Pathol. 29*: 413–449.
8. Andreason, A. P. (1958). *Myelofibrosis.* Munksgaard, Copenhagen.
9. Lennert, K., Nagaik, and Schwarze, E.-W. (1975). Patho-anatomical features of the bone marrow. *Clin. Haemat. 4*: 331–351.
10. Favre, M., Croizat, P., and Guichard, A. (1934). La myelose aleucemique megacaryocytaire. *Ann. Méd. 35*: 1–43.
11. Hittmair, A. (1944). Megakaryocytenleukämie und Osteomyelosklerose, ein einheitliches Krankheitsgeschen. *Klin. Wchnschr. 23*: 71–73.
12. Vaughan, J., and Harrison, C. V. (1939). Leuco-erythroblastic anaemia and myelosclerosis. *J. Pathol. Bactiol. 48*: 338–352.
13. Sanerkin, N. G. (1964). Stromal changes in leukaemia and related bone marrow proliferations. *J. Clin. Pathol. 17*: 541–547.

14. Mettier, S. R., and Rusk, G. Y. (1937). Fibrosis of the bone marrow (myelofibrosis) associated with a leukaemoid blood picture. Report of two cases. *Am. J. Pathol. 13*: 377–388.
15. Roberts, B. E., Miles, D. W., and Woods, C. G. (1969). Polycythaemia vera and myelosclerosis: A bone marrow study. *Brit. J. Haematol. 16*: 75–85.
16. Hutt, M. S. R., Pinniger, J. L., and Wetherley-Mein, G. (1953). The myeloproliferative disorders with special reference to myelofibrosis. *Blood 8*: 295–314.
17. Burston, J., and Pinniger, J. P. (1963). The reticular content of bone marrow in haematological disorders. *Br. J. Haematol. 9*: 172–183.
18. Bentley, S. A., Alabaster, O., and Foidart, J. M. (1981). Collagen heterogeneity in normal human bone marrow. *Br. J. Haematol. 48*: 287–291.
19. Irving, E. A., and Tomlin, S. G. (1954). Collagen, reticulum and their argyrophil properties. *Proc. Roy. Soc. B 142*: 113–125.
20. Charron, D., Robert, L., Couty, M.-C., and Binet, J.-L. (1979). Biochemical and histological analysis of bone marrow collagen in myelofibrosis. *Br. J. Haematol. 41*: 151–161.
21. Robert, L., and Dische, Z. (1963). Analysis of a sulfated sialofucoglycosaminogalactomanosidoglycan from corneal stroma. *Biochem. Biophys. Res. Commun. 10*: 209–214.
22. Fietzek, P. P., and Kuhn, K. (1976). The primary structure of collagen. *Int. Rev. Connec. Tissue Res. 7*: 1–60.
23. Castro-Malaspina, H., and Moore, M. A. S. (1982). Pathophysiological mechanisms operating in the development of myelofibrosis: Role of megakaryocytes. *Nouv. Rev. Fr. Hematol. 24*: 221–226.
24. Korst, D. R., Clatanoff, D. V., and Schilling, R. F. (1956). On myelofibrosis. *Arch. Int. Med. 97*: 169–183.
25. Linman, J. W., and Bethell, F. H. (1957). Agnogenic myeloid metaplasia. Its natural history and present day management. *Am. J. Med. 22*: 107–122.
26. Bouroncle, B. A., and Doan, C. A. (1962). Myelofibrosis: clinical, hematologic and pathologic study of 110 patients. *Am. J. Med. Sci. 243*: 697–715.
27. Ward, H. P., and Block, M. H. (1971). The natural history of agnogenic myeloid metaplasia (AMM) and a critical evaluation of its relationship with the myeloproliferative syndrome. *Medicine (Baltimore) 50*: 357–420.
28. Takácsi-Nagy, L., and Graf, F. (1975). Definition, clinical features and diagnosis of myelofibrosis. *Clin. Haematol. 4*: 291–308.
29. Varki, A., Lottenberg, R., Griffith, R., and Reinhard, E. (1983). The syndrome of idiopathic myelofibrosis: a clinicopathologic review with emphasis on the prognostic variables predicting survival. *Medicine (Baltimore) 62*: 353–371.

30. Lewis, S. M. (1983). The spleen–mysteries solved and unresolved. *Clin. Haematol. 12*: 363–373.
31. Goldman, J. M., and Nolasco, I. (1983). The spleen in myeloproliferative disorders. *Clin. Haematol. 12*: 505–516.
32. Njoku, O. S., Lewis, S. M., Catovsky, D., and Gordon-Smith, E. C. (1983). Anaemia in myelofibrosis: Its value in prognosis. *Br. J. Haematol. 54*: 79–89.
33. Block, M., and Jacobson, L. O. (1950). Myeloid metaplasia. *J. Am. Med. Assn. 143*: 1390–1396.
34. Dameshek, W. (1951). Some speculations on the myeloproliferative syndromes. *Blood 6*: 372–375.
35. Modan, B., and Lillienfeld, A. M. (1965). Polycythemia vera and leukaemia. The role of radiation treatment. *Medicine (Baltimore) 44*: 305–344.
36. Szur, L., and Lewis, S. M. (1966). The haematological complications of polycythaemia vera and its treatment with radioactive phosphorus. *Br. J. Radiol. 39*: 122–130.
37. Tubiana, M., Flamant, R., Attie, E., and Hayat, M. (1968). A study of hematological complications occurring in patients with polycythemia vera treated with P-32. *Blood 32*: 536–548.
38. Silverstein, M. N. (1974). Post-polycythemic myeloid metaplasia. *Arch. Intern. Med. 134*: 113–116.
39. Modan, B. (1975). Inter-relationship between polycythaemia vera, leukaemia and myeloid metaplasia. *Clin. Haematol. 4*: 427–439.
40. Silverstein, M. N. (1976). The evolution into and the treatment of late stage polcythemia vera. *Semin. Haematol. 13*: 79–84.
41. Wasserman, L. R., Balcerzak, S. P., Berk, P. D., Berlin, N. I. et al. (1981). Influence of therapy on causes of death in polycythemia vera. *Trans. Assoc. Am. Physic.* 30–38.
42. Pettit, J. E., Lewis, S. M., and Goolden, A. W. G. (1978). Polycythaemia vera–transformation to myelofibrosis and subsequent reversal. *Scand. J. Haematol. 20*: 63–69.
43. Pettit, J. E., Lewis, S. M., and Nicholas, A. W. (1979). Transitional myeloproliferative disorder. *Br. J. Haematol. 43*: 167–184.
44. Lewis, S. M., and Szur, L. (1963). Malignant myelosclerosis. *Br. Med. J. iii*: 472–477.
45. Castleman, B., and McNeely, B. V. (1966). Weekly clinico-pathological exercises: Case 24–1966. *New Engl. J. Med. 274*: 1200–1208.
46. Lubin, J., Rozen, S., and Rywlin, A. M. (1976). Malignant myelosclerosis. *Arch. Int. Med. 136*: 141–145.
47. Bird, T., and Proctor, S. J. (1977). Malignant myelosclerosis: Myeloproliferative disorder or leukemia. *Am. J. Clin. Pathol. 67*: 512–520.

48. Fabich, D. R., and Raich, P. C. (1977). Acute myelofibrosis: A report of three cases. *Am. J. Clin. Pathol. 67*: 334–338.
49. Ali, N. O., and James, W. D. (1979). Malignant myelosclerosis (acute myelofibrosis). Report of two cases following cytotoxic therapy. *Cancer 43*: 1211–1215.
50. Bearman, R. M., Pangalis, G. A., and Rappaport, H. (1979). Acute ("malignant") myelosclerosis. *Cancer 43*: 279–293.
51. Efrati, P., Nir, E., Yaari, A., Berrebi, A., Kaplan, H., and Dvilanski, A. (1979). Myeloproliferative disorders terminating in acute micromegakaryoblastic leukaemia. *Br. J. Haematol. 43*: 79–86.
52. Den Ottolander, G. J., te Velde, J., Brederoo, P., Geraedts, J. P. M., Slee, P. H. T. J., Willemze, R., Zwaan, F. E., Haak, H. L., Muller, H. P., and Bieger, R. (1979). Megakaryoblastic leukaemia (acute myelofibrosis): a report of three cases. *Br. J. Haematol. 42*: 9–20.
53. Bain, B. J., Catovsky, D., O'Brien, M., Prentice, G. H., Lawlor, E., Kumaran, T. O., McCann, S. R., Matutes, E., and Galton, D. A. G. (1981). Megakaryoblastic leukemia presenting as acute myelofibrosis—a study of four cases with the platelet peroxidase reaction. *Blood 58*: 206–213.
54. Burke, J. M., and Ross, R. (1977). Collagen synthesis by monkey arterial smooth muscle cells during proliferation and quiescence in culture. *Exp. Cell Res. 107*: 387–395.
55. Ross, R., and Vogel, A. (1978). The platelet-derived growth factor. *Cell 14*: 203–210.
56. Groopman, J. E. (1980). The pathogenesis of myelofibrosis in myeloproliferative disorders. *Ann. Int. Med. 92*: 847–858.
57. Jacobson, R. J., Salo, A., and Fialkow, P. J. (1978). Agnogenic myeloid metaplasia, a clonal proliferation of hematopoietic stem cells with secondary myelofibrosis. *Blood 51*: 189–194.
58. Lewis, C. M., and Pegrum, G. D. (1977). Immune complexes in myeloproliferative disorders. *Lancet ii*: 1151–1153.
59. Caligaris Cappio, F., Vigliani, R., Novarino, A., Camussi, G., Campana, D., and Gavosto, F. (1981). Idiopathic myelofibrosis: A possible role for immune-complexes in the pathogenesis of bone marrow fibrosis. *Br. J. Haematol. 49*: 17–21.
60. Rondeau, E., Solal-Celigny, P., Dhermy, D., Vroclans, M., Brousse, N., Bernard, J. F., and Boivin, P. (1983). Immune disorders in agnogenic myeloid metaplasia: relations to myelofibrosis. *Br. J. Haematol. 53*: 467–475.

2

Clinical and Hematological Aspects of Chronic Myelofibrosis

COLIN G. GEARY
University Department of Haematology, The Royal Infirmary, Manchester, England

INTRODUCTION

There are difficulties in defining "chronic myelofibrosis" (PMF) and "agnogenic myeloid metaplasia" (AMM) as clinical entities, because these terms are also used, with a pathological connotation, to describe features found in a wide spectrum of myeloproliferative disease (see Chapter 1). The clinical diagnosis of PMF is most frequently applied to a group of patients whose normal bone marrow stroma is replaced by dense bands of collageneous fibrous connective tissue, or even membranous bone, (osteomyelosclerosis, OMS) and in whom no underlying systemic disorder can be identified. Very frequently, such patients also exhibit two other characteristic features: myeloid metaplasia in spleen and liver, and a leukoerythroblastic blood picture. However, histologists also recognize increased stromal reticulin as a form of myelofibrosis and, indeed, there seems to be no compelling reason to separate the two types on biochemical or biophysical grounds (1). Within the context of chronic myeloproliferative disease (MPD), patients exhibiting the other clinical and hematological features of PMF may show only reticulin fibrosis in a hyperplastic marrow on trephine biopsy; in one major study, such patients accounted for a quarter of the total (2). Although it is possible to impose arbitrary criteria defining the degree and extent of fibrosis before allotting the patient the clinical diagnosis of PMF (3), the situation is confused because these have not always been adopted in earlier studies of the natural history of the disease.

Early proponents of the concept of myeloproliferative disease considered that fibroblastic proliferation, like that of hematopoietic cells, resulted from a postulated stimulation of pluripotent stem cells (4). This concept, although still of interest in comprehending the overlapping features of individual diseases, must be fundamentally modified in the light of later work defining the autonomous nature of blood cell proliferation in polycythemia vera (PV) and other members of the group. Moreover, as discussed elsewhere in this book, there is evidence from cytogenetic and other cell-marker studies that marrow fibrosis, though it may dominate the histological picture, is reactive to the underlying hematopoietic neoplasia, and in particular to the presence of abnormal megakaryocytes, and not part of that process. However, only a relatively small number of patients with MPD have been analyzed in this way: in particular the clonality of blood cell proliferation in PMF has not been proved in all cases, so it is possible that some have a different pathogenesis: for example an aberrant immune process (5). This might be consistent with the rare but well-documented spontaneous or therapy-related remissions that have been associated with complete disappearance of bone marrow fibrosis (6, 7). Recent work suggests that agents that cause dissolution of collagen fibrosis may also improve hematopoietic function (8).

The spectrum of myeloproliferative disease in which marrow fibrosis may be conspicuous is shown in Figure 1. It might be argued that, if fibrosis is an epiphenomenon associated with hemopoietic dysplasia, it is inappropriate to use the term as a definitive clinical diagnosis. However, it is convenient to retain it for practical reasons to describe a group of patients with reasonably distinctive clinico-pathological associations, and in whom the natural history is fairly predictable (2, 7, 9): in particular, evolution into acute leukemia is comparatively late and uncommon. The group is a heterogeneous one, nevertheless, and merges imperceptibly into other hemopoietic dysplasias, some of which also have a chronic clinical course ("undifferentiated" or "atypical" MPD) (3, 10), and often show hyperplastic marrows with megakaryocytic hyperplasia, and a group more appropriately included under the generic title of preleukemic myelodysplasias (11) (see Chapter 8). When bone marrow fibrosis occurs in the second type of case, it is characteristically out of proportion to the degree of myeloid metaplasia, and the clinical course is often rapidly fatal (see Chapter 7).

The physician may be able to recognize more than one clinical picture in relation to a particular point in the spectrum of myeloproliferative disease il-

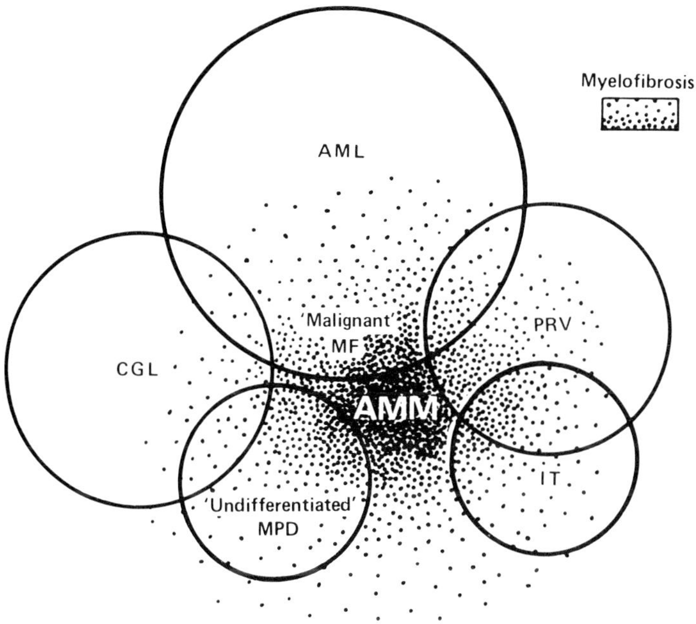

Figure 1 Myelofibrosis in the myeloproliferative syndrome. Myelofibrosis occurs in a wide spectrum of myeloproliferative disease, but in PMF and AMM it dominates the histological picture. Megakaryocytic hyperplasia is often conspicuous in these cases and the term "megakaryocytic myelosis" is used synonymously by some workers (18). The term "undifferentiated MPD" has been assigned to cases with predominantly cellular marrows but conspicuous myeloid metaplasia; these are often distinguishable clinically from "acute" or "malignant" myelofibrosis. AMM = Agnogenic myeloid metaplasia, AML = acute myeloblastic leukemia, IT = idiopathic thrombocythemia.

lustrated in Figure 1. For example cases transitional between PV and PMF may be identified as end-stage or "burnt out" disease with progressive marrow failure, but some have a stable or only slowly progressive disease with a very different natural history.

INCIDENCE AND EPIDEMIOLOGY

There have been few epidemiological studies of PMF. Woodliffe and Douigan (12) found an overall annual incidence of 0.6/100,000 with a M:F ratio of 2:1 in western Australia; Ward and Block (2) found the disease to be about one-quarter as common as chronic granulocytic leukemia (CGL) in Denver.

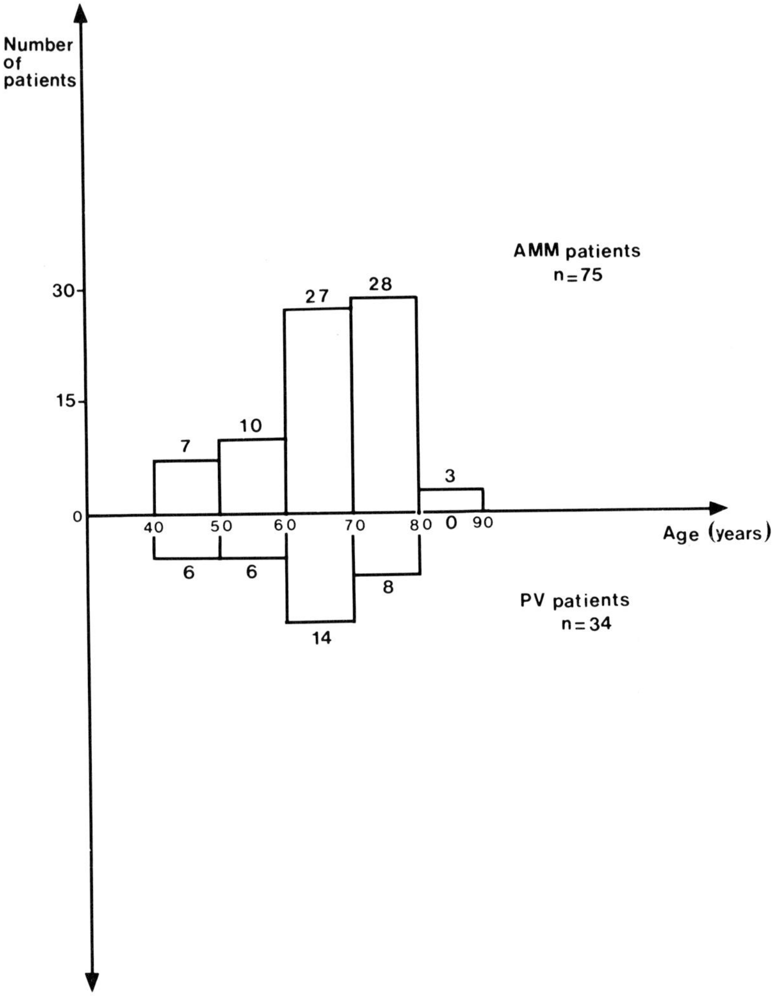

Figure 2 Age distribution of 67 cases of PMF at diagnosis [from Rondeau et al. (Ref. 15), reproduced by permission]. The smaller number of PV patients may represent differences in referral patterns to this particular clinic.

Some interesting racial factors have been reported. PMF is relatively more common in caucasians born in Europe who have later emigrated to Australia than in other ethnic groups resident in that country (12), and is also said to be rare in blacks, and in Spanish Americans (2). It occurs in the Japanese, and was one of the bone marrow disorders encountered among atom bomb victims (13, 14). In common with other chronic MPD, cases classified as PMF occur predominantly in middle aged and elderly people. The age distribution found in one large French clinic (15) is shown in Figure 2. Bouroncle and Doan (9) found a sharp reversal in the usual M:F preponderance within the 60–70 year age group, but this has not been identified by other workers. Experience in our Manchester clinic suggests that, like PV and CGL, PMF is commoner in men than women at all ages. A disease resembling PMF or OMS has been described in children (16–18), but it seems likely that some of the documented cases would now be diagnosed as megakaryoblastic leukemia or preleukemic myelodysplasia. The uncertain time of onset and insidious course usually frustrate attempts to associate the incidence of the disease with environmental factors; however, myeloid metaplasia occasionally follows benzene exposure, and Silverstein (19) has suggested a possible link between industrial solvents and the development of AMM or PMF.

CLINICAL FEATURES AT DIAGNOSIS

PMF is a progressive but usually very chronic disorder, the clinical diagnosis being preceded by a long symptom-free interval, which may last for many years: according to Block (20), in an average case, for two-thirds of the natural history of the disease. During this period there is gradually increasing myeloid metaplasia with progressive enlargement of the spleen and, sometimes, the liver. Ward and Block (2) suggest that the size of the spleen at diagnosis gives some indication of the duration of the disease; on the basis of observations made in untreated patients, these workers estimated that the disease had been present for 1 year for each centimeter that the spleen extended below the costal margin. Many patients are relatively asymptomatic at diagnosis, which is often made incidentally, following a routine blood count, or because the physician detects splenomegaly during routine physical examination. Ward and Block (2) found that, even with splenomegaly exceeding 16 cm, one-quarter of their patients volunteered no symptoms.

When symptoms do occur, they may be divided into three main groups: (a) those due to splenic enlargement, (b) those associated with the metabolic consequences of the underlying myeloproliferative disorder, and (c) those due to bone-marrow failure. The patient may notice a dragging sensation in the left abdomen due to splenomegaly, or notice changes in gastrointestinal motility due to pressure; a small minority have more severe pain due to perisplenitis. Metabolic symptoms are less conspicuous than in other myeloproliferative disorders, but weight loss is not uncommon and occasional patients complain of itching, sweating, or fever. Hyperuricemia may lead to gout or renal colic; Silverstein (19) noted acute gout in 6% of his patients, whereas Ward and Block (2) found it relatively more frequently (16%) in those presenting with massive splenomegaly.

As in other chronic MPD, fatigue is a fairly frequent complaint and that does not necessarily correlate with the hemoglobin level; other symptoms due to anemia occur in about 50% of patients, and become more common in older subjects. Less than 10% of patients, present with a serious bleeding diathesis, but skin bruising may occur, and rarely, gastrointestinal hemorrhage due to an associated portal hypertension may be the presenting symptom. Persistent bone pain is occasionally a feature, but is more likely to accompany later leukemic transformation.

Physical Examination

In the great majority of patients, the only significant finding at diagnosis is splenomegaly (2, 9, 19), which is almost always present. The spleen may become enormous, extending into the pelvis and across the midline. In one series (19), one-third of patients had such massive splenomegaly at diagnosis; it is characteristically very firm, and the notch is easily felt. Weights of 5 kg or more have been recorded at operation. Absence of clinical splenomegaly does not exclude the diagnosis of PMF: in such cases the spleen may be demonstrable by scintigraphy. As the disease progresses, the spleen becomes palpable, but rarely splenic atrophy may follow splenic arterial thrombosis in patients with marked thrombocytosis.

Hepatomegaly is less common at diagnosis, occurring in between 50 and 75% of patients (19); it is characteristically less conspicuous than splenomegaly, although gross hepatomegaly may occur after splenectomy. About 20% of patients have hepatomegaly greater than 6 cm at diagnosis. Signs of liver failure are rare at this stage, but may mark the terminal phases of the disease. Ascites is usually associated with portal hypertension and parenchymal liver failure and, again, tends to be a late feature; rarely, implants of myeloid tissue in the peritoneal cavity cause ascites (21). Lymphadenopathy is unusual, though Rosenthal and Moloney (22) reported a surprisingly high incidence of 22% in their series. Although the spleen and liver are the organs characteristically involved by myeloid metaplasia in PMF, pathological examination in advanced cases shows that extramedullary hematopoiesis can occur in practically any organ that is the site of blood formation in fetal life, with the possible exception of the thymus (2, 23). Occasionally this can give rise to unusual clinical presentations. For example, masses of myeloid tissue may occur in the lymph nodes, kidneys, lungs, pleura, gastrointestinal tract, peritoneum, retroperitoneal space, dura, skin, and breast (2). Rarely, multiple masses of extramedullary myeloid tissue may cause diagnostic confusion (24).

There are well-documented cases of involvement of the central nervous system (CNS) by myeloid tissue. Sometimes, the mass arises from bone but impinges from an extradural site on brain or, more commonly, spinal cord; thus, paraplegia or raised intracranial pressure may occur with focal neurological signs. However, dural and intracranial deposits also occur. An interesting case of CNS involvement has recently been described by Cornfield and his colleagues (25) in a patient with long-standing AMM who developed a progressive dementia. Computed tomography (CT) scanning demonstrated multiple intracranial masses, and their nature was confirmed by scanning with ^{52}Fe. A biopsy was thus avoided and marked improvement followed cranial irradiation to the masses. The subject of CNS involvement in PMF has recently been reviewed by Ligumski et al. (26). Ward and Block (2) give a comprehensive bibliography of clinical case reports describing unusual sites of myeloid metaplasia in this disease.

LABORATORY FEATURES

Morphological changes occur in the blood before the onset of anemia in PMF, although there is no pathognomonic blood picture in PMF analagous to that occurring in CGL or PV. Even anemia is not invariable, although most patients show a modest decline in the hemoglobin level; Njoku et al. (27) found some correlation between the hemoglobin level and age at diagnosis. The blood counts found at diagnosis in two large series are shown in Table 1; it is clear that the "proliferative" features of the marrow disorder are not always reflected in the peripheral blood picture, a significant number of patients having pancytopenia. A leukoerythroblastic blood picture is not invariable, although a careful search of the blood film will usually reveal an occasional normoblast: nevertheless, Silverstein (19) found a leukoerythroblastic reaction in 96% of his cases. Anisocytosis and poikilocytosis are also the rule, but they may be relatively inconspicuous and the classical "tear-shaped" poikilocytes may be quite sparse. Macrocytosis is also sometimes noted, particularly when residual marrow shows dyserythropoiesis, but the ovalocytosis seen in preleukemic myelodysplasia is rarely a feature. Deeply basophilic macrocytes,

Table 1 Blood Counts Found at Diagnosis in Two Large Series of Patients with Myelofibrosis and Myeloid Metaplasia

	Ward and Block (1971) (2)		Njoku et al. (1983) (27)	
	45 Cases	Percent	44 Cases	Percent
Hemoglobin (g/dl)	Mean 10.6		>10	54
			<10	46
Reticulocytes	–		<2%	32
			>2%	68
White blood cells (10^9/l)	4	13		20
	4–10	31		39
	10	55		41
Platelets (10^9/liter)	"Low"	22	<100	23
	"Normal"	49	100–500	59
	"High"	29	>500	8

representing "erythropoietin stress" are often seen in PMF. The cause of the extreme aniso- and poikilocytosis seen in many cases is not clear but may reflect abnormal hemopoiesis in extramedullary sites as well as disorganized bone marrow stroma. Red cell morphology sometimes improves after splenectomy (though normoblastemia tends to increase).

The causes of anemia in PMF are complex and are summarized in Table 2. Although bone marrow erythropoiesis is often reduced, there are extramedullary factors that contribute significantly to the pathogenesis of the anemia. Sequestration of red cells by the enlarged spleen and plasma volume expansion are the most important of these and are discussed in more detail below. In the marrow itself, ineffective erythropoiesis, recognizable morphologically, and by iron kinetic studies, is a frequent feature; this may be complicated by secondary folate deficiency, and occasionally ring sideroblasts are seen in advanced disease. Rarely, sideroblastic anemia may be the precursor of PMF, and interestingly, response to vitamin B_6 in PMF has been reported (28). However, iron deficiency due to gastrointestinal blood loss is commonly seen in patients with portal hypertension.

Most patients with PMF have a moderate reduction in the red cell life span (29, 30), and this is due both to defective erythropoiesis and hypersplenism: a positive red cell antiglobulin test is occasionally found (31). A red cell

Table 2 Causes of Anemia in Myelofibrosis

Bone marrow failure
quantitative
dyserythropoiesis (includes megaloblastosis, sideroblastosis, PNH–abnormality, etc.)
Plasma volume expansion
Splenic sequestration of red cells
Hemolysis
Intrinsic red cell defect, hypersplenism, ?red cell sensitization
Blood loss
platelet and/or coagulation deficiencies and defects
portal hypertension, etc.

defect similar to that found in paroxysmal nocturnal hemoglobinuria (PNH) was originally described by Lewis and his colleagues (32) in PMF and may occur in as many as 50% of patients (33). An abnormal sucrose lysis test is more common than a positive acidified serum lysis test. Although of interest as evidence of a clonal marrow disorder, it probably has only the same significance in PMF as in other patients with acquired dyserythropoietic anemias; occasionally a patient with PMF has transformed into the clinical picture of PNH, with intravascular hemolysis and hemoglobinuria (34). Rarely, acquired hemoglobin H disease may complicate PMF (35). Other intrinsic red cell defects known to occur in dyserythropoietic and preleukemic disorders are not characteristic of IMF but erythrocyte glucose-6-phosphate dehydrogenase (G6PD) and 6-phosphogluronic acid dehydrogenase levels tend to be increased. Serum lactic dehydrogenase levels are sometimes elevated in PMF, and, again, probably reflect dyserythropoiesis in medullary and extramedullary sites (2).

Leukocytes in PMF

A modest leukocytosis is usual at diagnosis though normal or even low counts are not uncommon (Table 1). In contrast to the hemoglobin and platelet counts, there is a tendency for the granulocyte count to rise as the disease progresses, although Silverstein found that 16% of his patients had persistent neutropenia (19). An occasional myelocyte may be seen even in patients with normal white blood cells; although a more pronounced shift to the left, with up to 10% of blast cells, is seen later in the disease and especially in patients with higher counts, the characteristic "dromedary" differential profile of CGL, with approximately equal numbers of myelocytes and segmented neutrophils, is absent. Bone marrow and blood basophilia may be present and hyperhistaminemia has been correlated with certain systemic symptoms, such as pruritis (36); it is not certain whether increasing basophilia has the same significance as in CGL–viz. a feature of impending acute leukemic transformation. Serum and urinary lysozyme levels may be slightly raised in PMF (37), but the high values seen in certain myelodysplastic diseases are not encountered, at least in the early stages. This may be a useful diagnostic pointer (38).

The leukocyte alkaline phosphatase (LAP) score is typically normal or raised in PMF; in general, patients with the highest granulocyte counts have the highest LAP score (39, 40); the neutrophils may show other metabolic features of the activated state, e.g., increased adherence (41). Total vitamin B_{12} binding capacity is usually raised in PMF, but rarely to the levels found in untreated CGL, reflecting the smaller granulocyte mass. No distinctive morphological changes occur in the granulocytes on conventional microscopy, but dysplastic features, affecting particularly the nucleus, have been described on ultrastructural examination (42). The appearance of Pelger cells, or of monocytosis suggest a preleukemic myelodysplasia. A number of functional defects in the granulocytes of PMF patients have been described (43, 44), and these may be relevant to the high incidence of infection in the later stages of the disease. Lymphopenia is occasionally found in PMF, but no distinctive changes in lymphocyte morphology are described.

Serum uric acid levels are frequently raised in PMF (2), particularly in patients with extensive myeloid metaplasia, and especially those with a previous history of PV. Raised serum alkaline phosphatase levels are found in a proportion of cases and probably reflect bone rather than hepatic disease (2).

Platelets in IMF

There is wide variation in the platelet count at diagnosis (Table 1). Patients with very high counts tend to have less marked splenomegaly and some may overlap with essential thrombocythemia. Giant platelets are often conspicuous, and sometimes megakaryocytic fragments, or even megakaryoblasts, are identified in the blood. The latter are thought to indicate extramedullary sites of thrombopoiesis and may be useful in distinguishing myeloproliferative disease from secondary thrombocythemia. Many ultrastructural abnormalities have been described in the platelets of patients with PMF (45, 46); there are sparse granules, whereas the microtubules are disorganized and membrane abnormalities are often present. Megakaryocytes in PMF often show considerable variation in size, and morphology (47).

Platelet function is defective in up to 50% of patients with PMF but it is not always possible to correlate in vitro tests with the clinical picture, and no pathognomonic constellation of abnormalities has emerged. Curiously, the larger platelets, which are metabolically the most active in normal individuals, seem to be particularly defective in PMF (48). In patients who show both a bleeding and thrombotic tendency, there are probably multiple abnormalities of platelet function, separately affecting hemostasis and the microvasculature (10). Abnormalities are similar to those occurring in essential (idiopathic) thrombocythemia, and include diminished response to aggregating agents such as serotonin, epinephrine, and adenosine diphosphate (ADP). Responses to collagen and thrombin have been reported normal in some patients (49, 50), but abnormal in others with defective release of platelet factor III (51).

Although platelet adhesiveness is often reduced, spontaneous aggregation also occurs; this effect can be abolished by small doses of aspirin. In fact, thrombosis has been shown to be less frequent in chronic MPD than might be expected from the level of the platelet count (52); conversely, bleeding may occur with a platelet count higher than in other clinical situations. The latter is particularly important in relation to gastrointestinal or cerebral hemorrhage, or when splenectomy is contemplated in PMF. The bleeding time was found to be prolonged in 20% of one series of patients with PMF (19); this clinical abnormality correlated best with the severity of thrombocytopenia. Splenomegaly has profound effects on the distribution of the platelet mass in the body; in patients with gross splenomegaly, as much as 90% of the platelet mass may be sequestered in the spleen. Weinfeld et al. (48) showed the platelet life span to be reduced in PMF; in spite of a considerable increase in production from medullary and extramedullary sources, the patient is often thrombocytopenic. These earlier kinetic studies, using ^{51}Cr as a label, have been confirmed using indium-labeled platelets (52a).

Coagulation Abnormalities

A variety of coagulation abnormalities have been described in PMF. The subject has been reviewed by Silverstein (19), who found 29 out of 39 patients to have abnormal prothrombin times. Gilbert and Wasserman (53) also found abnormal prothrombin times in 37% of 19 patients with PMF. In some cases, Factor V levels have been diminished and there has been evidence of fibrinolysis, with low fibrinogen levels and raised titers of fibrin degradation products

(19). Hepatic dysfunction (see below) may set the scene for both coagulation factor deficiency and activation of the fibrinolytic system, with chronic, often subclinical, disseminated intravascular coagulation. Rarely, a circulating anticoagulant has been documented, and this may reflect immunological disturbance.

Immunological Abnormalities

There has been much interest in clinical and laboratory evidence of immune disorders in PMF in recent years (54, 55), but it remains uncertain whether these are related to the etiology of the disease or epiphenomena of disordered stem cell growth. Thus, both hyperglobulinemia and hypoglobulinemia (55a) have been reported in comparable patient groups; rarely, a monoclonal protein may occur (19). Immune complexes in leukocytes were demonstrated in several patients with PMF by Lewis and Pegrum (54), who suggested that they might indicate a favorable response to immunosuppressive therapy. In a recent study, Rondeau and his colleagues (15) found that many patients with PMF show laboratory evidence of disturbed immunological function. 75% of 67 patients showed one or more of the following abnormalities: serum antinuclear and antismooth muscle antibodies, rheumatoid factor, a polyclonal increase in serum immunoglobulin levels, or a serum monoclonal component, a positive red cell antiglobulin test, and an anti-I autoantibody. There was no relationship with clinical features, such as age, duration of disease, or spleen size. Interestingly, such abnormalities were found only one-third as frequently in patients with PV. The authors suggest that this high incidence of autoimmune phenomena indicates a lymphoid abnormality consequent upon stem cell dysfunction and, like Lewis and Pegrum, postulate immune mechanisms in the pathogenesis of PMF. Bone marrow interstitial immunoglobulin deposits have been demonstrated in PMF, but not in osteomyelosclerosis due to carcinoma (56). A chronic inflammatory infiltrate characterized by lymphocytes, plasma cells, and mastocytes is sometimes seen in myelofibrotic marrows (57). Rarely, a disease resembling PMF has been found in the context of a well-defined autoimmune disorder like systemic lupus erythematosis (58). It has been suggested that depressed or abnormal splenic function in chronic myeloproliferative disease might predispose to autoimmune reactions (15).

RADIOLOGICAL FEATURES OF PMF AND OMS

The classical radiological features of OMS are patchy increase in bone density and obliteration of the corticomedullary junction. The association between

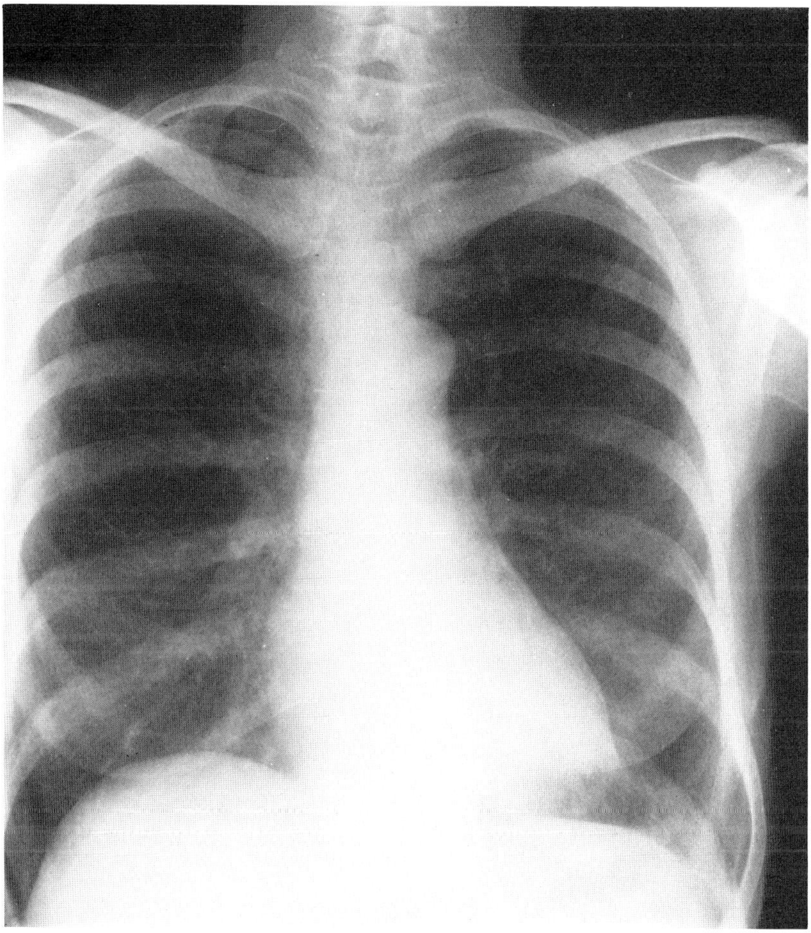

Figure 3 Early evidence of osteosclerosis in a chest radiograph. There is increased density of both clavicles, and the corticomedullary junction, particularly in the medial thirds of the bones, is poorly defined.

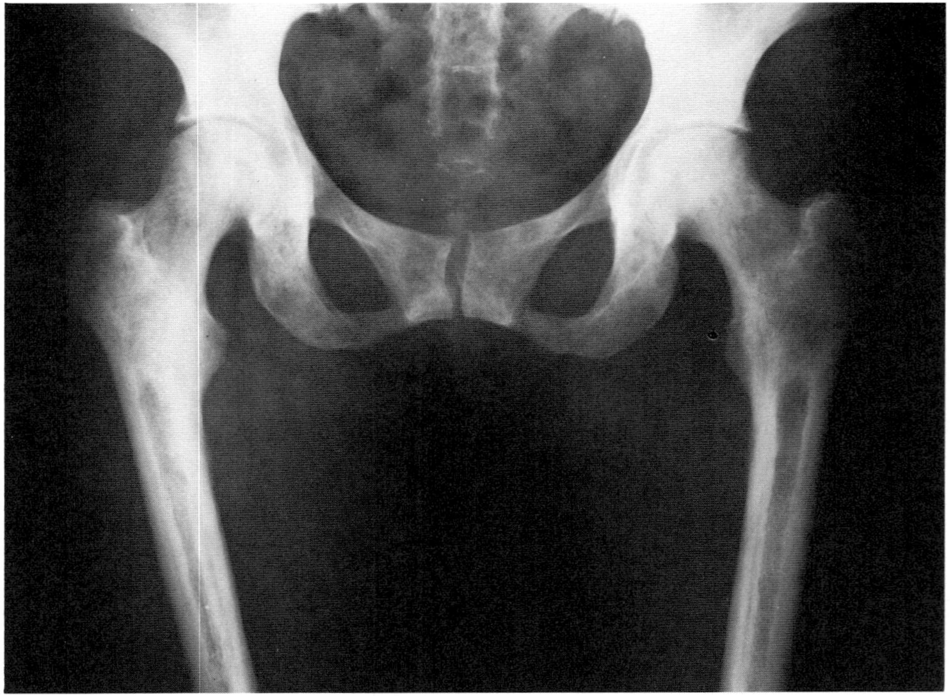

Figure 4 Advanced osteomyelosclerosis. There is generalized increase in bone density, and patchy loss of trabecular pattern. The irregularity of the corticomedullary junction in the femora is well shown. New endosteal bone is conspicuous in the upper third of the shafts. Note also the tendency of the osteosclerotic areas to symmetry; for example, in the medial aspects of the inferior pubic rami.

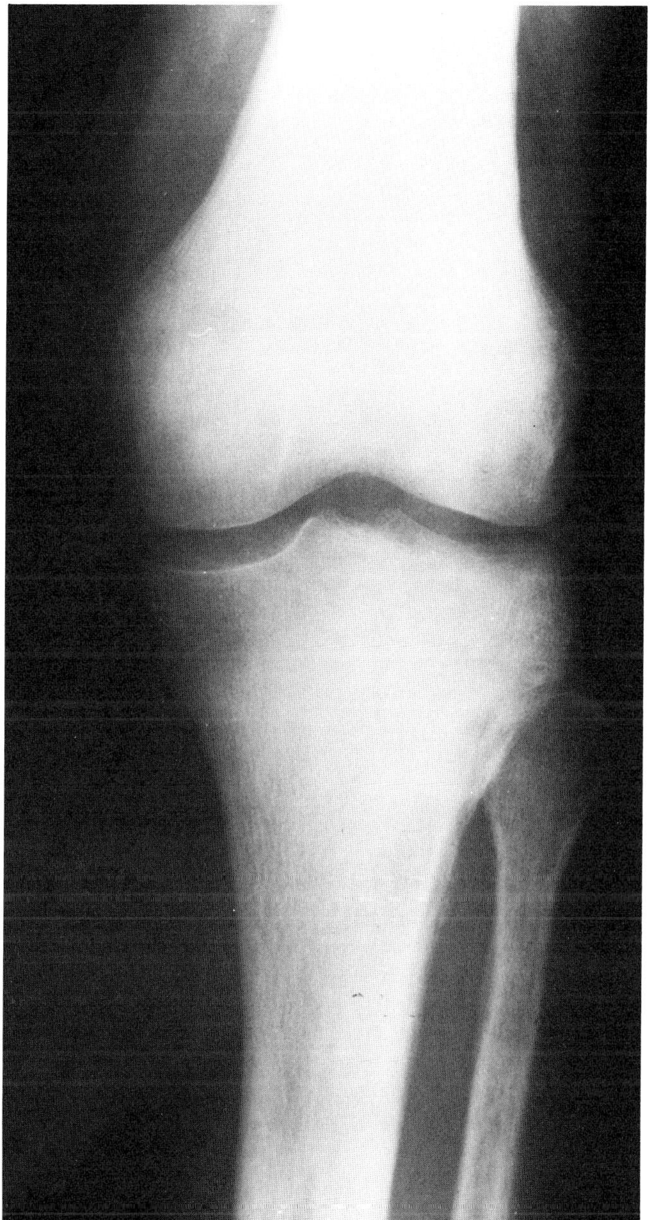

Figure 5 Periosteal reaction in PMF. There is new bone formation, particularly at the distal end of the femur, and also some loss of trabecular striation. (Courtesy of Dr. T. Patton.)

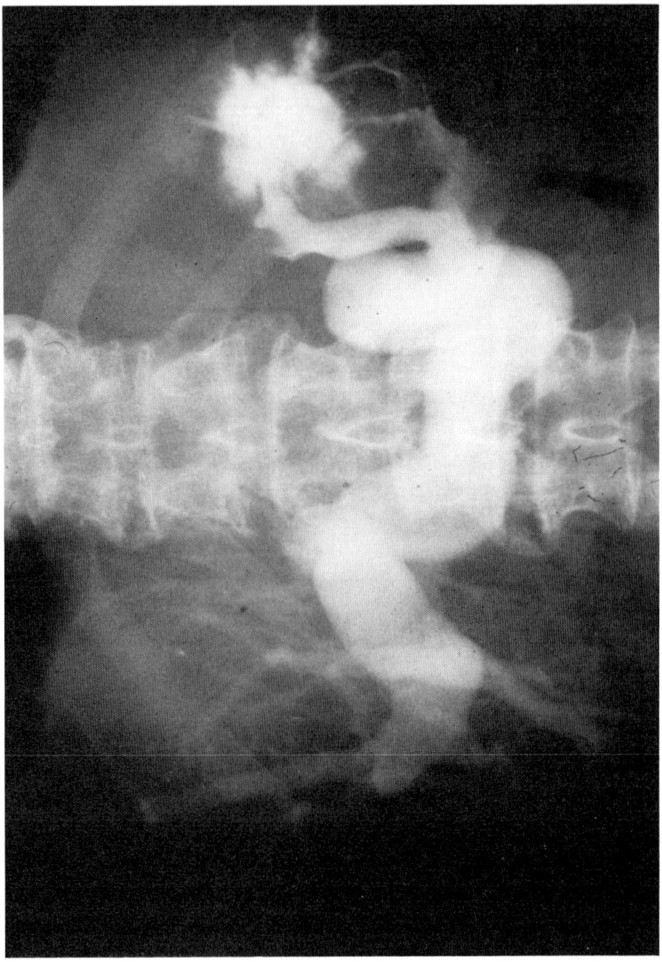

Figure 6 "Spleno-portagram" in a patient with portal hypertension complicating PMF. The dilated splenic and portal venous vessels are clearly shown. (Courtesy of Dr. R.C. Routledge.)

radiologically demonstrable osteomyelosclerosis and a leukoerythroblastic blood picture was the cardinal feature of the classic paper by Vaughan and Harrison (59). Laszlo (3) has pointed out that the frequency with which radiological abnormalities are documented in PMF and OMS depends on how the author has defined his patient material, and the extent of the skeletal examination; Ward and Block (2) found that 40% of their series of 45 patients had some evidence of osteosclerosis. Analysis of this series, and several smaller ones, led to an estimate that one-third of patients had sufficient osteosclerosis to be detectable by "casual inspection" of a chest x-ray (Fig. 3). The distribution of osteosclerosis in PMF is fairly characteristic, affecting the axial skeleton, and particularly the red marrow-containing bones, in the early stages. The ribs, clavicles, pelvis, and vertebral bodies are most commonly affected, but radiological abnormalities in the metaphyseal areas of the femur and humerus also occur (Figs. 4 and 5). The changes may be diffuse and widespread or patchy; in suspected cases, it is valuable to compare the radiograph with that from a normal individual of the same age and sex (60). There is, characteristically, increased density due to new bone deposition in the trabeculae ("ground-glass appearance") and also to endosteal cortical thickening; in the skull vault, increased density may be associated with disappearance of the diploic space. There may be narrowing of the medullary spaces of the long bones; irregular periosteal reactions near the ends of the long bones are an occasional feature (Fig. 6).

Myelofibrosis itself is not always associated with increased radiographic density; in some cases, areas of focal bone marrow hyperplasia and subsequent fibrosis leading to bone resorption may result in translucent areas (60) and loss of the usual trabecular pattern, although here loss of the demarcation between cortex and medulla is also seen. Pathological fractures are, however, very unusual. One characteristic feature of the bone changes in osteomyelosclerosis is a tendency to symmetry, in sharp distinction to those found, for example, in carcinomatosis or Paget's disease (61). Bone scintigraphy shows an increased medullary blood flow in PMF (62).

PORTAL HYPERTENSION IN PMF AND OMS

An important complication of PMF, and less commonly other chronic MPD, is portal hypertension, with or without hepatic cirrhosis. Many patients have abnormal liver function tests in the later stages of the disease. Some reviews suggest that portal hypertension occurs in as many as 20% of patients with PMF and OMS (3); Lennert found cirrhosis more frequently in patients with OMS (63). Recently, Ligumski and his colleagues (64) found clinical evidence of portal hypertension in 20 out of 37 cases of PMF studied. The most dramatic clinical picture is that associated with the Budd-Chiari syndrome, in which occlusion of the hepatic vein, or its major radicles, produces acute enlargement and failure of the liver, and ascites (65); in its most severe form, it is rapidly fatal, but chronic forms of the syndrome have been described. This "postsinusoidal" venous obstruction must be distinguished from "sinusoidal" obstruction, often secondary to infiltration of the liver by myeloid metaplasia, and "presinusoidal" obstruction, usually due to thrombosis in the portal vein or its branches (3, 66, 67). Although venous thrombosis is especially likely to occur in patients with high platelet counts, it is interesting that the PNH syndrome is also sometimes complicated in this way.

Periportal fibrosis also occurs in PMF; coexisting hepatic cirrhosis, alcoholism, or even hemosiderosis may be related to its pathogenesis. A type of hepatic cirrhosis peculiar to myelofibrotic patients has been postulated, but remains a doubtful entity (68). Kupffer cell hyperplasia is often conspicuous in the liver of PMF patients. In some patients, no organic obstruction to venous blood flow in the portal system can be detected, and myeloid metaplasia in the hepatic parenchyma may be inconspicuous (69). In these, there is dilation of the splenic and portal veins, and in some, though not all cases (66), blood flow is considerably increased, mainly as a result of splenic enlargement (Fig. 7). Increased blood flow through the splenoportal venous system does not invariably produce signs of portal hypertension; if there is no infiltration of the liver, there may be passive or active adjustment of vascular resistance so that even a massive increase of portal blood flow can be maintained without an abnormal increase in the pressure gradient across the portal-hepatic bed; thus, Rosenbaum et al. (67) reported hepatic blood flow that was three times normal in a patient with AMM who did not have portal hypertension. In others, "hyperkinetic" portal hypertension occurs; here the compliance of the liver is insufficient to accommodate the greatly increased blood flow. Ward and Block (2) have emphasized that myeloid metaplasia in the liver does not correlate well with the severity of portal hypertension.

If portal hypertension occurs, it is accompanied by the same clinical features as in other situations, e.g., esophageal and gastric varices, distended veins in the abdominal wall, and ascites. The factors involved in the pathogenesis of ascites and edema in patients with PMF are essentially similar to those occurring in cirrhosis, viz. portal hypertension leading to increased hydrostatic pressure in the preportal venous bed, salt retention due to hyperaldosteronism, and decreased colloid osmotic pressure if there is hypoalbuminemia (67). The role of lymphatic obstruction—a common contributory factor in other forms of liver disease—in the ascites of PMF and AMM is

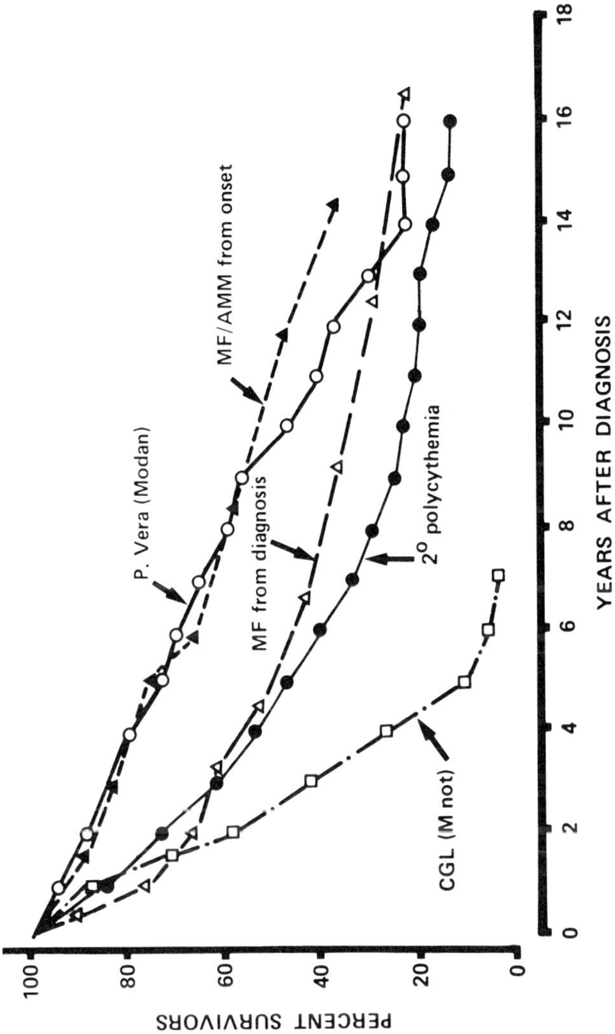

Figure 7 Survival times in various types of chronic myeloproliferative disease. [From Ward and Block (Ref. 2) with permission.]

unknown. The expansion of the portal vascular space is now believed to be an important factor in causing the increase in plasma volume that occurs in many patients with PMF (see p. 128).

PROGNOSIS OF PMF

Patients with this disease show a remarkable variability in their natural history. Ward and Block (2) suggested that there were two subsets of patients when prognosis was considered; however, the total duration of the disease includes a long preclinical phase in the majority of patients. The average survival from diagnosis ranges from 24 months to about 5 years in published series. Silverstein and Rubin found that approximately half their series of 169 patients survived 5 years but noted a better survivorship in the patients who were asymptomatic at diagnosis; these authors also suggested that two prognostic groups could be defined. Bouroncle and Doan (9), analyzing 110 cases, found that only 8% of their patients survived more than 6 years. Nevertheless, there are anecdotal reports of survival of up to 40 years (18).

Various clinical and laboratory features have been reported to affect survival in PMF; these include age, presence of symptoms, hemoglobin and platelet counts, reticulocyte count, red cell survival, red cell volume, percentage incorporation of iron into red cells, and bone marrow histology (2, 19, 30, 70). Interestingly, although it has been suggested that massive splenomegaly indicates long-standing disease (2), the size of the spleen per se does not seem to correlate with subsequent survival, although plasma volume expansion, consequent upon splenic enlargement, is of predictive value (27). Hepatomegaly, was, however, found to be an important adverse prognostic pointer by Silverstein (19). Njoku and his colleagues (27) have recently suggested that a reliable prognostic index can be derived by analysis of the hemoglobin and reticulocyte count at diagnosis, patients with hemoglobins below 10 g/dl and reticulocyte counts below 2% having the worst prognosis with a median survival of only 1.7 years; by contrast patients with hemoglobin levels of more than 10 g/dl had median survivals in excess of 6 years.

The variability in the natural history of PMF makes it difficult to evaluate the effects of treatment, such as splenectomy, in the management of the disease. The most common causes of death in PMF are infection, particularly of the respiratory and renal tracts, cerebro- or cardiovascular disease, gastrointestinal bleeding, and acute leukemia. A small minority die of hepatic or renal failure. Silverstein (19) has drawn attention to the frequency with which widespread advanced degenerative vascular disease, and cardiac failure, are encountered in PMF; it must be remembered, however, that the disease occurs most frequently in that group of individuals in whom atherosclerosis is also common, namely middle-aged and elderly men. Interestingly, plasma cholesterol levels are often low in advanced PMF (41).

DIAGNOSIS OF PMF

There are two stages in the diagnosis of PMF (a), establishing that bone marrow fibrosis results from intrinsic marrow disease rather than some systemic disorder, and (b) the definition of PMF within the spectrum of chronic MPD. An emphasized above, PMF merges imperceptibly into the other members of the group, and it is sensible to use diagnostic criteria to define the disease. The American Polycythaemia Vera Study Group (3) has defined PMF as a clinical illness with splenomegaly, fibrosis involving more than one-third of the sectional area of an adequate bone marrow biopsy, a leukoerythroblastic blood picture, absence of an increased red cell mass, and absence of the Philadelphia chromosome on cytogenetic analysis, with systemic disorders excluded; criteria for the diagnosis of OMS are similar, except for the presence of sclerotic changes detected radiologically in axial skeleton or long bones. Careful clinical examination and microscopy of an adequate bone marrow trephine biopsy taken, if necessary, from more than one site are essential in distinguishing PMF from "secondary" marrow fibrosis with or without extramedullary erythropoiesis. The usual problem is to distinguish PMF from carcinoma or lymphoma with marrow involvement. It must be remembered that splenic myeloid metaplasia is frequently found at autopsy in many patients with carcinomatosis and marrow involvement. Nevertheless, splenomegaly is rarely as conspicuous as in PMF and there are frequently other clues, especially more pronounced metabolic symptoms, e.g., weight loss, fever, and cachexia, even if there are none specifically referable to a primary neoplasm. Although a leukoerythroblastic picture frequently occurs in this situation, the typical changes in red cell morphology that characterize PMF and OMS are rather less conspicuous in carcinoma. Among the lymphomata, leukemic reticuloendotheliosis, often associated with marked splenomegaly and pancytopenia, sometimes causes diagnostic difficulty. However, the marrow picture is characterized by heavy reticulin fibrosis rather than collagen fibrosis, and the characteristic "hairy cells" are usually seen in the blood. The distinction of PMF and OMS from the myelodysplastic syndromes is discussed in Chapter 8.

The absence of distinctive blood changes and bone marrow fibrosis should easily distinguish those patients who have substantial splenomegaly due to primary liver disease and portal hypertension. Gaucher's disease, tuberculosis, and histoplasmosis occasionally give rise to a picture simulating PMF. In the last two conditions, the relevant organisms may be demonstrated in marrow culture, or where applicable, in splenic aspirates; in perplexing cases, a chemotherapeutic trial may be justifiable. Although there is no doubt that tuberculosis can occasionally produce bone marrow fibrosis and a leukoerythroblastic blood picture (71, 72), in many of the published cases it seems likely that tuberculosis has complicated established myeloproliferative disease. In either context, the distribution and histology of the tuberculous lesions is unusual, and may be found only in the lymph nodes, liver, spleen, and bone marrow. An interesting rarity that occasionally produces a clinical and pathological picture closely resembling PMF is systemic mastocytosis (73): in these cases, the usual skin manifestations and hyperheparinemia may be absent, but patchy osteoporosis, as well as fibrosis and sclerosis are characteristic. Portal hypertension also occurs, but the typical leukoerythroblastic blood picture of PMF seems to be unusual.

Differential Diagnosis Within the Chronic MPD: Transitional Forms

As marrow fibrosis occurs throughout the spectrum of MPD, inevitably diagnostic difficulties arise. There are clinicopathological descriptions of patients who, although showing some of the features of classical PMF, also exhibit those of other members of the group. This overlapping picture is seen most frequently in relation to PV. Approximately one-sixth of patients with classical PV eventually develop the clinical picture of PMF with progressive enlargement of the spleen and functional evidence of bone marrow failure; extensive collagen fibrosis occurs in some, whereas in others, the marrow remains cellular with only reticulin fibrosis. This syndrome has been called postpolycythemic myeloid metaplasia (PPMM) by Silverstein (74) and "spent polycythemia" by earlier workers. According to Wasserman, all patients with PV are liable to develop this syndrome if they live long enough (75). Its clinical course is more rapid than that of PMF arising de novo; survival is shorter and the risks of hemorrhage and leukemia are higher than in the latter group. It is postulated that the use of myelosuppressive agents might be related to the later development of this syndrome (74, 76). However, Szur (77), and Pettit et al. (78) have described a form of myeloproliferative disease intermediate between PV and PMF, which, although it shows features of the latter disease, may be potentially reversible, at least as regards bone marrow function. These patients often present with polycythemic blood counts, but also have a leukoerythroblastic blood picture and usually extensive reticulin or even collagen fibrosis in the marrow. Splenic myeloid metaplasia is present and may dominate the clinical picture. These patients differ from those with

PPMM in the sense that the inexorable progression into myelofibrosis with increasing anemia and thrombocytopenia need not occur if the correct treatment is chosen. According to Pettit and his colleagues (78), myelosuppressive therapy should be avoided, even when the patient is still in a polycythemic phase; ^{32}P, in particular, is a bone-seeking element and may encourage further extra medullary erythropoiesis. Splenectomy may be particularly appropriate. These patients do not, strictly speaking, have "masked polycythemia" because when anemia supervenes the red cell mass may be within normal limits. The remarkable chronicity of this type of case is seen in Figure 8. The rise in hemoglobin that occurs in these cases after splenectomy is often very slow, suggesting that the correction of a dilutional anemia is not the only factor responsible, that extramedullary erythropoiesis is not necessarily beneficial, and that the spleen may in some circumstances compete with, or inhibit, marrow function.

Another transitional form of MPD that sometimes gives rise to diagnostic difficulty is one intermediate between CGL and PMF. There are no problems in distinguishing classical CGL from PMF on examination of the blood picture and bone marrow histology. Bone marrow reticulin, however, increases during the evolution of the disease and becomes particularly conspicuous before the onset of blastic transformation; collagen fibrosis can also occur at this stage with refractory splenomegaly and a leukoerythroblastic blood picture. Nevertheless, the presence of the Philadelphia chromosome and the previous history indicate the correct diagnosis in such cases. Clough et al. (79), in a survey of bone marrow trephine biopsies from 45 cases of CGL, found that a small number *presented* with most if not all the features of PMF or even OMS; had not the Philadelphia chromosome been demonstrable in blood or marrow, these patients would have been diagnosed as PMF. One interesting feature was that they had higher LAP scores than usually found in chronic-phase CGL. The cellular trilineage of extramedullary hemopoiesis, characteristic of PMF, may occasionally be present in the spleen, though granulocytic hyperplasia often persists.

The literature contains a number of reports of "Philadelphia positive" PMF (80–83). According to Ward and Block (2), CGL only complicates PMF if mutagenic agents have been used to treat the earlier myeloproliferative disease, but other reports suggest that a transitional form of disease does exist. Thus, Georgii and his colleagues (5) performed combined histological and cytogenetic studies in 33 patients clinically diagnosed as PMF and OMS, including 11 in acute leukemic transformation, using a special technique to obtain marrow material for cytogenetic analysis from bone marrow trephines. Of these 33, 22 showed the Philadelphia chromosome. The authors suggest

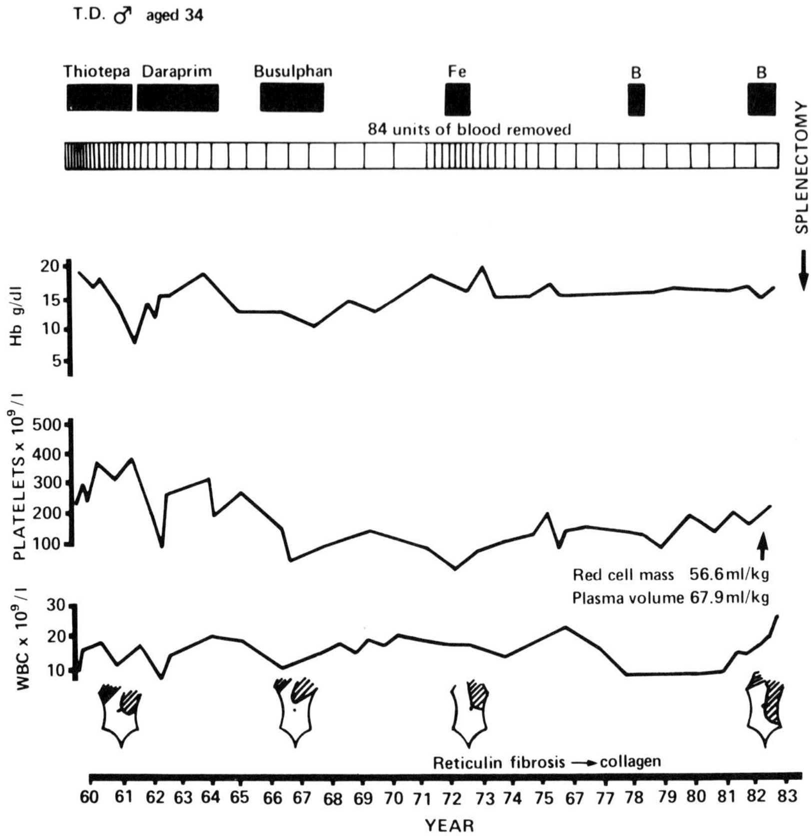

Figure 8 A 23-year survival in a male patient with transitional myeloproliferative disorder. This patient was polycythemic for much of his course, but showed myeloid metaplasia from the outset. Occasional normoblasts were seen in the blood smear at the time of diagnosis and later he had a frankly leukoerythroblastic blood picture. The spleen weighed 5 kg at operation, and showed extensive myeloid metaplasia, but negligible fibrosis. There has been a modest thrombocytosis since splenectomy, but the hemoglobin is now stable. The marrow histology now shows widespread collagen fibrosis.

that some cases of PMF are really "occult" CGL with a fibrotic marrow; failure to recognize them in the past was related to technical difficulties in establishing the chromosomal status of marrow cells. However, the proliferative pattern of circulating stem cells is different in the two diseases. Idiopathic thrombocythemia (IT) is usually associated with only slight splenomegaly and myeloid metaplasia; the red cell changes of IMF are absent. Nevertheless, a small proportion of these patients eventually evolve into a picture indistinguishable from PMF. It is of some interest, however, in the context of the role of megakaryocytes in the pathogenesis of marrow fibrosis, that many of these patients have only trivial reticulin fibrosis at diagnosis.

Acute Leukemia in PMF

There are wide variations in the reported incidence of acute leukemia in PMF and OMS; Burkhardt (18) found it less commonly in the latter syndrome. It has been argued that leukemic transformation is not part of the natural history of the disease but may result from treatment (2). However, Emberger and his colleagues (84) collected from the literature 30 cases of PMF and AMM in which acute leukemia evolved in patients with little or no myelosuppressive therapy. Moreover, the fact that some patients show cytogenetic abnormalities similar to those found in acute nonlymphocytic leukemia and preleukemic myelodysplasias suggest an affinity between at least some cases of PMF and acute leukemia (5). Bentley et al. (85), reviewing the literature on PMF, found that the average incidence of acute leukemia was about 8%; the incidence is higher in patients with previous PV. Acute leukemia occurs more frequently in males and usually within 5 years of the original diagnosis of PMF, but it has been recorded as early as 6 months and as late as 14 years. The great majority of the reported cases have been acute nonlymphocytic (myeloblastic and myelomonocytic) leukemia, but megakaryoblastic and even lymphoblastic leukemia (86) have been described. Except possibly in the last type, the disease often leads a rapidly progressive course and is resistant to usual chemotherapeutic regimens. There are occasional reports of "histiocytic" and other solid tumors arising in the marrows of patients with PMF and OMS (18).

Clinically, transformation into acute leukemia may be suspected by the following: rapid increase in spleen size, lymphadenopathy, onset of bone pain, loss of weight or sudden onset of fever or sweating; hematologically, there is often a sudden fall in the hemoglobin and platelet count in a previously stable case. A sudden increase in peripheral blood blastemia should alert suspicion, although an exaggerated leukoerythroblastic response may also occur as a response to infection or hemorrhage. Sometimes there is a change in the morphology of the blast cells, e.g., appearance of cytoplasmic vacuoles, monocytoid forms, or Auer rods. Marrow aspirates are usually difficult to obtain, but on trephine biopsy, sheets of blast cells are sometimes visible. Neutrophil myeloperoxidase activity may decline (87). Other laboratory features that are indicative of blastic transformation are a fall in a previously high LAP score, an increase in serum lysozyme concentration (38), an abrupt change in the proliferative characteristics of progenitor cells colony-forming units, granulocyte macrophage (CFU–GM), in the peripheral blood and a deterioration in the bone marrow scanning patterns using ^{52}Fe, with apparent erythroid hypoplasia in previously active medullary and extramedullary sites (85).

Splenomegaly in PMF and AMM

Myeloid metaplasia in PMF and AMM is thought to result from the "seeding" of potential extramedullary sites for hemopoiesis by a monoclonal population of stem cells or their progeny, presumably originating from medullary sources. However, it is not clear why some patients have such extreme splenic myeloid metaplasia. As discussed above, there is some correlation between splenic size and duration of disease, but massive splenomegaly may coexist with good marrow function.

Whatever the explanation, it is clear that substantial splenomegaly, when present, dominates the blood picture in PMF. Although the term "hypersplenism" is often used loosely to denote the influence of the spleen in this condition, the mechanisms by which cytopenias are produced in the chronic MPD are complex (88). Thrombocytopenia is due in large part to sequestration of platelets; on the other hand, there is only a small splenic pool of granulocytes even in massive splenomegaly. Thus, granulocytopenia, when present, seems to relate to failing marrow function or vascular margination.

The hematocrit is influenced in several ways. A large spleen is associated with a slow transit time of red cells through the pulp, with increased irreversible trapping of abnormal cells in the splenic cords (88), so that an element of splenic hemolysis is superimposed on an erythrocyte population already physically and metabolically abnormal as a result of dyshemopoiesis. In addition, the splenic red cell pool is much increased in myeloid metaplasia; for a given degree of splenomegaly, red cell pooling in this disease is often greater than in other causes of congestive or infiltrative enlargement (89). Although in slow dynamic equilibrium with the circulating red cell mass, as much as one-third or even more of the total red cell volume may effectively be sequestered in the spleen, (Fig. 9) so that the venous hematocrit is proportionately

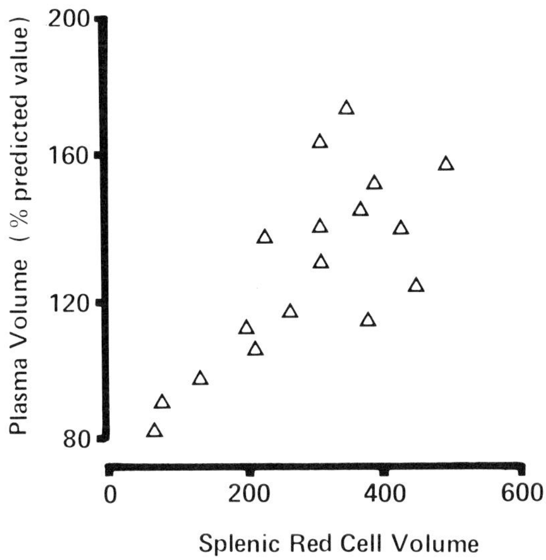

Figure 9 Correlation of splenic red cell pool with expansion of plasma volume in patients with PMF. [From Njoku et al. (Ref. 27), reproduced by permission.]

reduced. This large splenic red cell pool itself contributes to the increased size of the organ. Isotopic labeling of red cells may nevertheless show that the total body red cell mass is normal or even increased, especially in patients with massive splenomegaly.

Another important effect of splenomegaly is expansion of the plasma volume. This occurs in most conditions associated with enlarged spleens, irrespective of the underlying pathology (90, 91). Expansion of total blood volume occurs approximately pari passu with the degree of splenomegaly. In many cases, the increase in plasma volume is much more than can be ascribed to an increased anatomical vascular space created by an enlarging spleen. The spleen acts, functionally if not anatomically, as an arteriovenous shunt, so that blood flow into the portal venous system increases (92). In turn, there is often a chronic increase in portal venous pressure which leads to an expansion of the splanchnic vasculature (see p. 32). An increased total blood volume is required to fill this increased intravascular space. In patients without hematological disease, this demand will be met by a proportional increase in red cells and plasma, so that the venous hematocrit is not grossly abnormal, unless there are other factors, such as malnutrition or hyperglobulinemia. However, in patients with seriously impaired bone marrow function, demand for increased volume has to be met proportionally more by expansion of the plasma compartment.

Plasma volume is normally controlled, inter alia, by osmo- or baroceptors in the great veins and kidney. Hess (93) has suggested a train of events resulting from a chronic expansion of the portal vascular space; these include diminished renal arterial perfusion, increased renin secretion, and salt and water retention (Fig. 10). In patients with good liver function, this increase in plasma volume is accommodated by an increased rate of albumin synthesis, so that many patients with PMF do not have conspicuous peripheral edema. Later, deteriorating liver function may be associated with edema and ascites. Anemia per se does not seem to play a role in plasma volume expansion. In PMF, as in some other diseases associated with massive splenomegaly, there is sometimes an increased metabolic rate that is associated with vasodilatation and decreased peripheral resistance. These effects exacerbate the hemodynamic changes caused by the flow-induced portal hypertension (93). Portal pressure decreases after splenectomy, but plasma volume may take some weeks to return to normal and remains elevated in some cases. This may be due to residual portal obstruction in the liver, but in others the reason is not clear. Identification of any anatomical site of portal obstruction is of course important when splenectomy is contemplated in PMF.

Although the spleen has been regarded as an important hemopoietic organ in late-stage PMF, experience shows that the hemoglobin rarely falls after splenectomy in this disease (29); indeed, there are reports of improved marrow erythropoiesis after splenectomy (94). The advantages of reduction in plasma volume, and abolition of splenic pooling of red cells, outweigh any loss of hematopoietic function. Recent work has confirmed these clinical impressions; thus, Njoku and his colleagues (27) have shown that the total red cell mass correlates best with residual medullary hemopoiesis and not with the extent of extramedullary hemopoiesis, which is often ineffective (95). Plasma volume expansion seems to correlate inversely with prognosis; the most likely explanation is that patients with the largest plasma volume have the least good residual marrow function. Splenomegaly per se does not correlate with prognosis, since even large spleens may coexist with reasonably good medullary hemopoiesis; in this case, plasma volume expansion may be less marked.

These observations suggest that, even in advanced PMF, residual medullary function is critical in determining the red cell mass.

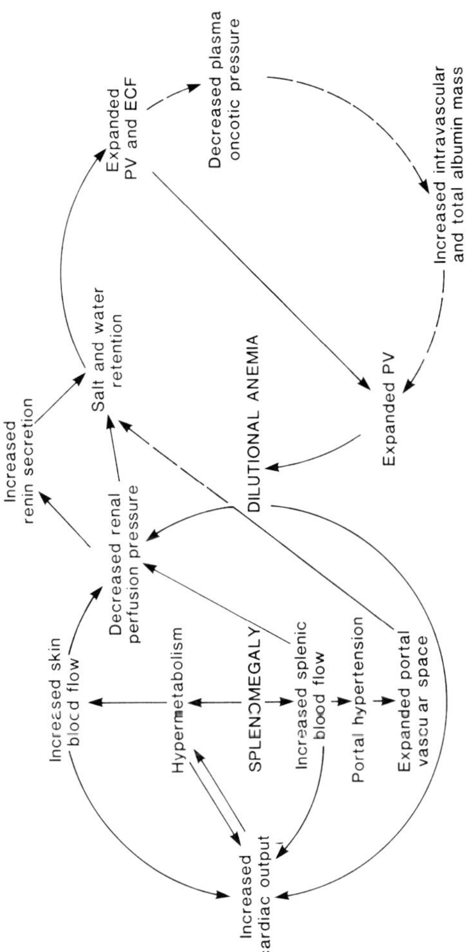

Figure 10 A possible mechanism of plasma volume expansion in patients with massive splenomegaly, leading to dilutional anemia. In addition to the hemodynamic results of portal hypertension, the hypermetabolism found in some patients with MPD may be a contributory factor (see text). [From Hess et al. (Ref. 93), reproduced from *Blood* by permission.]

REFERENCES

1. Prockop, D. J., Kivitikko, K. I., Tuderman, L., and Gunzman, N. A. (1979). The biosynthesis of collagen and its disorders. *N. Engl. J. Med. 301*: 13–23.
2. Ward, H. P., and Block, M. H. (1971). The natural history of agnogenic myeloid metaplasia and a critical evaluation of its relationship with the myeloproliferative syndrome. *Medicine 50*: 357–420.
3. Laszlo, J. (1975). Myeloproliferative disorders (MPD): Myelofibrosis, Myelosclerosis, Extramedullary Hematopoiesis, Undifferentiated MPD, and Hemorrhagic Thrombocythaemia. *Semin. Hemat. 12*: 75–98.
4. Dameshek, W. (editorial). (1951). Some speculations on the myeloproliferative syndromes. *Blood 6*: 372–375.
5. Georgii, A., Thiele, J., and Vykoupil, K. F. (1980). Osteomyelofibrosis: a histological and cytogenetic study on core biopsies of the Bone Marrow. *Virch. Arch. A. Path. Anat. and Histol. 389*: 269–286.
6. Tobin, M. S. (1975). Clinical considerations and treatment. In *Dahlem Workshop on Myelofibrosis–Osteosclerosis Syndrome.* Edited R. Burkhardt, C. L. Conley, K. Lennert, and others, Oxford, Pergamon Press, p. 247.
7. Shreiner, D. P. Spontaneous hematologic remission in agnogenic myeloid metaplasia. *Am. J. Med. 60*: 1014–1018.
8. Arlet, P. L., Nicodeme, R., Adoue, D., Lanagain-Fournier, Delsol, G., LeTallec, Y. (1984). Clinical Evidence for 1,25 hydroxycholecalciferol action in myelofibrosis. *Lancet i*: 1013–1014.
9. Bouroncle, B. A., and Doan, C. A. (1962). Myelofibrosis–clinical, hematologic and pathologic study of 110 patients. *Am. J. Med. Sci. 243*: 697–715.
10. Wetherley-Mein, G., and Pearson, T. C. (1982). The myeloproliferative disorders. In *Blood and its Disorders,* 2nd edition. Edited by R. M. Hardisty and D. J. Weatherall, Oxford, Blackwell, p. 1269–1316.
11. Lichtman, M. A. (1983). Hemopoietic stem cell disorders: Classification. In *Hematology*, 3rd edition. Edited by W. J. Williams, E. Beutler, A. J. Erslev, M. A. Lichtman, New York, McGraw Hill, pp. 144–150.
12. Woodliffe, H. J., and Douigan, L. (1974). Myelofibrosis: Incidence and prevalence in Western Australia (1960–1969). An epidemiological study of 64 cases. In *Dahlem Workshop on Myelofibrosis–Osteosclerosis Syndrome,* Oxford, Pergamon Press, p. 288.
13. Anderson, R. E., Hoshino, R., and Yamamoto, T. (1964). Myelofibrosis with myeloid metaplasia in survivors of the atomic bomb in Hiroshima. *Ann. Intern. Med. 60*: 1–18.
14. Block, M. H. Incidence of acute leukaemia and myelofibrosis in Japanese Survivors of the atom-bomb explosions. *Proc. XVII Congress International Society for Haematology,* Paris, p. 879.

15. Rondeau, E., Solal-Celigny, P., Dhermy, D., Vroclans, M., Brousse, N., Bernard, J. F., and Boivin, P. (1983). Immune disorders in agnogenic myeloid metaplasia: relations to myelofibrosis. *Br. J. Haematol. 53*: 467–475.
16. Tobin, M. S., Than, C., and Argano, S. A. P. (1969). Myelofibrosis in pediatric age group. *N.Y. St. J. Med. 69*: 1080–1083.
17. Nagai, K., Sugiyama, Y., Isono, Y., and Yoshida, K. (1969). An autopsy case of primary osteomyelosclerosis in a 6-year old girl. *Acta Pathol. Jap. 19*: 81–93.
18. Burkhardt, R., Bartl, R., Beil, E., et al. (1975). Review of literature and histomorphology of myelofibrosis–osteosclerosis syndrome. In *Dahlem Workshop on Myelofibrosis–Osteosclerosis Syndrome*. Edited by R. Burkhardt, C. L. Conley, and K. Lennert, and others, Oxford, Pergamon Press, pp. 18–19.
19. Silverstein, M. N. (1975). *Agnogenic Myeloid Metaplasia.* Publishing Sciences Group, Acton.
20. Block, M. (1975). Phylogenetic and embryological basis of myeloid metaplasia. In *Dahlem Workshop on Myelofibrosis–Osteosclerosis Syndrome.* Edited by R. Burkhardt, C. L. Conley, K. Lennert, and others, Oxford, Pergamon Press, pp. 105–125.
21. Gorshein, D., and Brauer, M. H. (1969). Ascites in myeloid metaplasia due to ectopic peritoneal implantation. *Cancer (Philadelphia) 33*: 1408–1412.
22. Rosenthal, D. S., and Moloney, W. C. (1969). Myeloid metaplasia. *Postgrad. Med. 45*: 136–142.
23. Beck, W. S. (1982). In *Hematology,* 3rd edition. Edited by W. S. Beck, London, MIT Press, p. 1.
24. Aach, R., and Kissane, J. (1971). Myelofibrosis with unusual neurologic abnormalities. *Am. J. Med. 51*: 799–811.
25. Cornfield, D. B., Shipkin, P., Alavi, A., Becker, J., and Peyster, R. (1983). Intracranial myeloid metaplasia: Diagnosis by C.T. and Fe^{52} scans and treatment by cranial irradiation. *Am. J. Hematol. 15*: 273–278.
26. Ligumski, M., Polliack, A., Benbassat, J. (1978). Myeloid metaplasia of the central nervous system in patients with myelofibrosis and agnogenic myeloid metaplasia. Report of 3 cases and review of the literature. *Am. J. Med. Sci. 275*: 99–103.
27. Njoku, O. S., Lewis, S. M., Catovsky, D., and Gordon-Smith, E. C. Anaemia in myelofibrosis: Its value in prognosis. *Br. J. Haematol. 54*: 79–89.
28. Roger, R. A., Mulder, N. H., Nieweg, H. O. (1978). Response to pyridoxine hydrochloride in refractory anemia due to myelofibrosis. *Am. J. Med. 65*: 655–660.

29. Milner, G. R., Geary, C. G., Wadsworth, L. D., and Doss, A. (1973). Erythrokinetic studies as a guide to the value of splenectomy in primary myeloid metaplasia. *Br. J. Haematol. 25*: 467–484.
30. Najean, Y., Cacchione, R., Castro-Malaspina, H., and Dresch, C. (1978). Erythrokinetic studies in myelofibrosis: Their significance for prognosis. *Br. J. Haematol. 40*: 205–217.
31. Hasselbach, H., Berild, D., and Hansen, O. P. (1984). Red cell sensitisation in myelofibrosis. *Scand. J. Haematol. 32*: 179–181.
32. Lewis, S. M., Pettit, J. E., Tattersall, M. H. N., et al. (1971). Myelosclerosis and paroxysmal haemoglobinuria. *Scand. J. Haematol. 8*: 451–460.
33. Kuo, C. Y., van Voolen, G. A., and Morrison, A. N. (1972). Primary and secondary myelofibrosis: Its relationship to "PNH-like defect." *Blood 40*: 875–880.
34. Hansen, S. E., and Killman, S. A. (1970). Paroxysmol nocturnal haemoglobinuria in myelofibrosis. *Blood 36*: 428–431.
35. Veer, A. (1979). Acquired hemoglobin H disease in idiopathic myelofibrosis. *Am. J. Hematol. 6*: 99.
36. Gilbert, H. S., and Krauss, S. (1970). In *Myeloproliferative Disorders in Animals and Man.* Edited by W. J. Clarke, E. B. Howard, and P. L. Hackett. USAEC Division of Technical Information, p. 429.
37. Hansen, N. E., and Anderson, V. Lysozyme activity in human neutrophilic granulocytes. *Br. J. Haematol. 24*: 613–623.
38. Skarin, A. T., Matsuo, Y., and Moloney, W. C. (1972). Muramidase in myeloproliferative disorders terminating in acute leukaemia. *Cancer (Philadelphia) 29*: 1336–1342.
39. Leonard, B. J., Israels, M. G. C., and Wilkinson, J. F. (1957). Myelosclerosis: A clinico-pathological study. *Q. J. Med. 26*: 131–145.
40. Mitus, W. J., Bergna, L. J., Mednicoff, I. B., and Dameshek, W. (1958). Alkaline phosphatase of mature neutrophils in chronic forms of the myeloproliferative syndrome. *Am. J. Clin. Pathol. 30*: 285–294.
41. Gilbert, H. S. (1984). Myelofibrosis revisited. In *Myelofibrosis and the Biology of Connective Tissue.* Edited by P. D. Berk, H. Castro-Malaspina, and L. R. Wasserman. New York, Alan R. Liss, Inc., pp. 3–17.
42. Bessis, M. (1972). In *Cellules de Sang.* Paris, Masson, pp. 685–695.
43. El-Maallem, H., and Fletcher, J. (1977). Impaired neutrophil function in myeloid metaplasia. *Br. J. Haematol. 37*: 323–335.
44. Marquetty, C., Labro-Bryskier, M. L., Perianin, A., and Hakin, J. (1984). Impaired metabolic activity of phagacytosing neutrophils in agnogenic osteomyelofibrosis with splenomegaly. *Am. J. Hematol. 16*: 243–254.
45. Maldonado, J. E., Pintado, T., and Pierre, R. V. (1974). Dysplastic platelets and circulating megakaryocytes in chronic myeloproliferative disorders. I. *Blood 73*: 797–809.

46. Zucker-Franklin, D. Ultrastructural studies of hematopoietic elements in relation to the myelofibrosis–osteosclerosis syndrome; megakaryocytes and platelets (MMM or MOS). In *Dahlem Workshop on Myelofibrosis–Osterosclerosis Syndrome,* pp. 127–143.
47. Maldonado, J. E., Pintado, T., and Pierre, R. V. (1974). Dysplastic platelets and circulating megakaryocytes in chronic myeloproliferative disorders. II. Ultrastructure of circulating megaykaryocytes. *Blood 43*: 811–829.
48. Weinfeld, A., Branehog, I., and Kutti, J. (1975). Platelets in the myeloproliferative syndromes. *Clin. Haematol. 4*: 373–392.
49. Inceman, S., and Tangun, Y. (1972). Platelet defects in the myeloproliferative disorders. *Ann. N.Y. Acad. Sci. 201*: 251–261.
50. Sultan, C., and Jeanneau, Y. (1973). Myeloproliferative disorders and platelet aggregation. In *Platelet Aggregation.* Edited by J. Caen, Masson et Cie, Paris, pp.
51. Neemeh, J. A., Bowie, E. J. W., Thompson, J. H., Didisheim, P., and Owen, C. A. (1972). Quantitation of platelet aggregation in myeloproliferative disorders. *Am. J. Clin. Pathol. 57*: 336.
52. Kessler, C. M., Klein, H. G., and Harlik, R. J. (1982). Uncontrolled thrombocytosis in chronic myeloproliferative disorders. *Br. J. Haematol. 50*: 157–167.
52a. Bautista, A. P., Buckler, P. W., Towler, H. M. A., Dawson, A. A., and Bennett, B. (1984). Measurement of platelet life span in normal subjects, and patients with myeloproliferative disease, with indium oxine labelled platelets. *Brit. J. Haematol. 58*: 679–687.
53. Gilbert, H. S., and Wasserman, L. R. (1964). Hemorrhage in surgery in myelofibrosis, multiple myeloma, leukaemia and lymphomas. *Ann. N.Y. Acad. Sci. 115*: 169–178.
54. Lewis, C. M., and Pegrum, G. D. (1978). Immune complexes in myelofibrosis; A possible guide to treatment. *Br. J. Haematol. 39*: 233–239.
55. Boivon, P., Bernard, J. F., Hakin, M., and Wroclans, M. (1974). Anomalies immunitaries au cours des splenomegalies myeloides. *Acta Haematol. 51*: 91–100.
55a. Selroos, O., Skrifvars, B., and Wasastjerna, C. (1973). Immunological deficiency in myelofibrosis. *Scand. J. Haematol. 11*: 307–313.
56. Barge, J., Slabodsky-Brousee, N., and Bernard, J. F. (1978). Histoimmunology of myelofibrosis: A study of 100 cases. *Biomedicine 29*: 73–75.
57. Caligaris-Cappio, F., Vigliani, R., Novarino, A., Camussi, G., Campara, D., and Gavosto, F. (1981). Idiopathic myelofibrosis: A possible role for immune complexes in the pathogenesis of bone marrow fibrosis. *Br. J. Haematol. 9*: 17–21.
58. Lau, K. S., and White, J. C. (1969). Myelosclerosis associated with sys-

temic lupus erythematosus in patients in West Malaysia. *J. Clin. Pathol. 22*: 433–438.
59. Vaughan, J. M., and Harrison, C. V. (1939). Leuco-erythroblastic anemia and myelosclerosis. *J. Pathol. Bacteriol. 48*: 339–352.
60. Murray, R. O. (1975). In *Textbook of Radiology,* 2nd edition. Edited by D. S. Sutton, London, Longman, p. 164.
61. Feldman, F. (1965). Myelosclerosis in agnogenic myeloid metaplasia. *Seminars in Roentgenology 9*: 195–207.
62. Van Dyke, D., Anger, H. O., Parker, H., McRae, J., Dobson, E. L., Yano, Y., Naets, J. P., and Linfoot, J. (1971). Markedly increased bone blood flow in myelofibrosis. *J. Nucl. Med. 12*: 506–512.
63. Lennert, K. (1975). Pathology and morphology of myelofibrosis. In *Dahlem Workshop on Myelofibrosis–Osteosclerosis syndrome.* Oxford, Pergamon Press, p. 239.
64. Ligumski, M., Polliack, A., and Benbassat, J. (1978). Myeloid metaplasia of the central nervous system in patients with myelofibrosis and agnogenic myeloid metaplasia. Report of 3 cases and review of the literature. *Am. J. Med. Sci. 275*: 99–103.
65. Schmidt, D., Ward, H. P., and Block, M. H. (1970). Agnogenic myeloid metaplasia and the Budd-Chiari syndrome. In *Myeloproliferative Syndromes of Animals and Man.* Edited by W. J. Clarke et al. Oak Ridge, Tennessee, USAES Division of Technical Information.
66. Shaldon, S., and Sherlock, S. (1962). Portal hypertension in the myeloproliferative syndromes and the reticuloses. *Am. J. Med. 32*: 758–764.
67. Rosenbaum, D. L., Murphy, G. W., and Swisher, S. N. (1966). Hemodynamic studies of the portal circulation in myeloid metaplasia. *Am. J. Med. 41*: 360–368.
68. Reubner, B. (1960). Myelosclerosis with serosal myeloid metaplasia and fatal liver involvement. *Ann. Int. Med. 53*: 1075–1088.
69. Blendis, L. M., Banks, D. C., Ramboer, C., and Williams, R. (1970). Spleen blood flow and splanchnic haemodynamics in blood dyscrasia and other splenomegalies. *Clin. Sci. 38*: 73–84.
70. Meytes, D., Katz, D., and Ramot, B. (1976). Prognostic parameters in myeloid metaplasia: Agnogenic vs post-polycythaemic. *Israel J. Med. Sci. 12*: 534–542.
71. Crail, H. W., Alt, H. L., and Nadler, W. H. (1948). Myelofibrosis associated with tuberculosis. *Blood 3*: 1426–1444.
72. Medd, W. E., and Hayhoe, F. G. J. Tuberculous miliary necrosis with pancytopenia. *Q. J. Med. (N.S.) 24*: 351–365.
73. Sawers, A. H., Davson, J., Braganza, J., and Geary, C. G. (1982). Systemic mastocytosis, myelofibrosis and portal hypertension. *J. Clin. Pathol. 35*: 617–619.
74. Silverstein, M. N. (1976). The evolution into and the treatment of late stage polycythemia vera. *Semin. Hematol. 13*: 189–194.

75. Wasserman, L. R. (1964). Polycythemia vera–its course and treatment. Relation to myeloid metaplasia and treatment. *Bull. N.Y. Acad. Med. Sci. 30*: 343-375.
76. Szur, L., and Lewis, S. M. (1966). The haematological complications of polycythaemia vera and treatment with radioactive phosphorus. *Br. J. Radiol. 39*: 122-130.
77. Szur, L. (1975). Clinical considerations and treatment. In *Dahlem Workshop on Myelofibrosis–Osterosclerosis Syndrome.* Edited by R. Burkhardt and others, Oxford, Pergamon Press, pp. 248-249.
78. Pettit, J. E., Lewis, S. M., and Nicholas, A. W. (1979). Transitional myeloproliferative disorder. *Br. J. Haematol. 43*: 167-184.
79. Clough, V., Geary, C. G., Hashmi, K., Davson, J., and Knowlson, T. (1979). Myelofibrosis in chronic granulocytic leukaemia. *Br. J. Haematol. 42*: 515-526.
80. Krauss, S. (1966). Chronic myelocytic leukaemia with features simulating myelofibrosis with myeloid metaplasia. *Cancer (Philadelphia) 19*: 1321-1332.
81. Smalley, R. V., Tassoni, E., and Durant, J. R. (1966). Chronic myeloid leukaemia and myelofibrosis. *Lancet 393.*
82. Galton, D. A. G. (1965). Problems in the management of the myeloproliferative states. *Series Haematologica 1*: 37-46.
83. Frey, I., and Siebner, H. (1968). Osteomyelofibrose mit Philadelphia (Ph') Chromosome. *Med. Welt 19*: 2274-2279.
84. Emberger, J. M., Wagner, A., and Izarn, P. (1969). La terminaison en leucémie aiguä de l'osteomyelofibrose avec métaplasie myéloide hépatosplénique. *Nouv. Rev. Fr. Hematol. 9*: 375-390.
85. Bentley, S. A., Murray, K. H., Lewis, S. M., and Roberts, P. D. (1977). Erythroid hypoplasia in myclofibrosis: A feature associated with blastic transformation. *Br. J. Haematol. 36*: 41-47.
86. Amjad, H., Gezer, S., Inove, S., Bollinger, R. O., Kaplan, J., Carson, S., and Bishop, C. R. (1980). Acute myelofibrosis terminating in an acute lymphoblastic leukaemia. *Cancer 46*: 615-618.
87. Rosenthal, D. S., and Moloney, W. C. (1977). Occurrence of acute leukaemia in myeloproliferative disorders. *Br. J. Haematol. 36*: 373-382.
88. Bowdler, A. J. (1983). Splenomegaly and hypersplenism. *Clin. Haematol. 12*: 467-488.
89. Pettit, J. E., Williams, E. D., Glass, H. I., Lewis, S. M., Szur, L., and Wicks, C. J. (1971). Studies of splenic function in the myeloproliferative disorders and generalised malignant lymphomas. *Br. J. Haematol. 20*: 575-586.
90. McFadzean, A. J. S., Todd, D., and Tsang, K. C. (1958). Observations on the anemia of cryptogenic splenomegaly II. Expansion of the plasma volume. *Blood 13*: 524-532.

91. Bowdler, A. J. Blood volume changes in patients with splenomegaly. *Transfusion 10*: 171–181.
92. Garnett, E. S., Goddard, B. A., Markby, D., and Webber, C. E. (1969). The spleen as an arterio-venous shunt. *Lancet i*: 386–388.
93. Hess, C. E., Ayers, C. R., Sandusky, W. R., Carpenter, M. A., Wetzel, R. A., and Mahler, D. N. (1976). Mechanism of dilutional anemia in massive splenomegaly. *Blood 47*: 629–644.
94. Wetherley-Mein, G., Jones, N. F., and Pullan, J. M. (1961). Effects of splenectomy on red cell production in myelofibrosis. *Br. Med. J. i*: 84–89.
95. Sjogren, V. (1978). Different composition of the erythropoietic tissue in bone marrow, spleen and liver in myelofibrosis. *Acta Haematol. 59*: 231–238.

3

Histology of Myelofibrosis and Osteomyelosclerosis

BERTHA FRISCH
Institute of Hematology, Ichilov Hospital, Tel Aviv Medical Centre, Tel Aviv, Israel

REINER BARTL
City Centre Hospital, University of Munich, Munich, West Germany

INTRODUCTION

The term "myelofibrosis" is taken to mean an increase in fine fibers (reticulin) in the bone marrow; "myelosclerosis" refers to an increase in coarse fibers (collagen); and "osteomyelosclerosis" is used when increased new bone formation–appositional, woven, or both–is also present. "Reticulin" and "collagen" fibers are well established morphologic terms, both of which refer to biochemically identical collagenous proteins.

The introduction of bone marrow biopsies in the investigation of patients with hematologic diseases in general (and not only in cases in which a dry tap is obtained on attempts at aspiration) has led to the more frequent recognition of fibrosis of the bone marrow in these disorders. In addition, sequential bone biopsies taken during periods of follow-up and monitoring of progression of various other disease processes have become available for retrospective analysis. It is now clear that fibrosis in the bone marrow may be divided into five major groups; as a consequence of (a) neoplastic myeloproliferative disorders (MPD), (b) neoplastic lymphoproliferative disorders (LPD), (c) extramedullary neoplasias growing in the bone marrow, (d) osseous disorders with augmented remodeling, such as hyperparathyroidism and Paget's disease of bone, and (e) inflammatory reactions due to toxins, drugs, immune complexes, and unidentified etiologic agents.

Most cases of fibrosis in the bone marrow fall into one of the first four groups, and very few, on careful examination, will today be found to belong to the last group, which includes cases of the so called "chronic idiopathic myelofibrosis" or any of its numerous synonyms (see Chapter 1).

These groups will be considered briefly and their similarities as well as their distinctive features (when present) will be given. However, the emphasis will be on myelofibrosis (MF) and osteomyelosclerosis (OMS), evolving as an integral part of the myeloproliferative diseases that will be considered in greater detail. The results given in this chapter are based on our own observations made on several thousand initial and sequential bone marrow biopsies.

PATIENTS AND METHODS

Bone marrow biopsies were taken of 3230 patients. Of these, 2529 patients were diagnosed by the established criteria as suffering from one of the MPD, or suspected hematologic disorders (including myelofibrosis) and a dry tap on aspiration. Bone biopsies were taken in 356 patients with tumors of lung, prostate, breast, or other organs; and in 88 patients with cytopenia(s) presumed to be due to inflammatory diseases, autoimmune states, or as a consequence of exposure to toxins. Informed consent was obtained after the procedure had been fully explained to the patients. Following local anesthesia, the biopsies were taken from the anterior or the posterior iliac crests. All biopsies were fixed, dehydrated, and embedded into plastic without prior decalcification and cut and stained as previously described (1-3). Giemsa stain was used for cytologic detail, Gomori's stain for reticulin fibers, Ladewig's stain and Toluidine Blue for calcified bone and osteoid, the periodic acid Schiff (PAS) reaction for glycoprotein, and the Prussian Blue stain for iron. In some cases, the biopsies were halved: one-half was fixed as above for plastic histology and one-half was frozen for enzyme and marker studies, after a small piece had been cut off for electron microscopy (EM). Sections cut in a cryostat were used for reactions with fluorescein isothiocyanate (FITC)-labeled antibodies. After fixation in glutaraldehyde, the piece for EM was dehydrated without prior decalcification and embedded in Spurr's medium. Thin sections were cut, stained with lead citrate and uranyl acetate, and viewed in a Zeiss EM 10. A number of clinical variables were registered for each patient at the time the biopsy was taken; 35 structural and 8 histomorphometric variables were evaluated for each biopsy; and these data were utilized for multivariate analysis by selected BMPD computer programs (2, 4).

GENERAL SURVEY OF MYELOFIBROSIS AND OSTEOMYELOSCLEROSIS (MF/OMS)

The normal bone marrow has only few fibers and these are found mainly in association with the trabecular bone surfaces and some blood vessels. The designation myelofibrosis itself refers only to the presence of increased connective tissue elements with no implications as to etiology. This fibrosis may occur in varying degrees of severity and has been roughly divided into three grades (Fig. 1). The basic disorders associated with bone marrow fibrosis are given in Figures 2 and 3a–h and Table 1, which includes only cases with grades II and III. A rapidly progressive form of bone marrow fibrosis (usually fatal) may also supervene in the course of various hematologic disorders, whether or not some degree of fibrosis was already present (Table 2). Myelofibrosis is initially due to an increase in reticulin fibers that, when progressive, leads to collagen fiber deposition and obliteration of the hematopoietic marrow. The types of collagen associated with components of the bone and bone marrow may be summarized as follows: type I with bone matrix, type III with the medial and adventitial coats of blood vessels and with the fibrosis of chronic inflammation, and type IV with sinusoidal endothelium and basement membranes. Examples are given in Figure 4. Myelofibrosis may or may not be accompanied by an increase in bone: appositional osteoblastic new bone formation onto the pre-existing trabeculae or woven, intramembranous bone within the marrow spaces. The extent of overall osseous increase is variable, and three grades are distinguished (Fig. 5). Correlations of the different fibrotic and osseous patterns with the basic disorders in the bone marrow

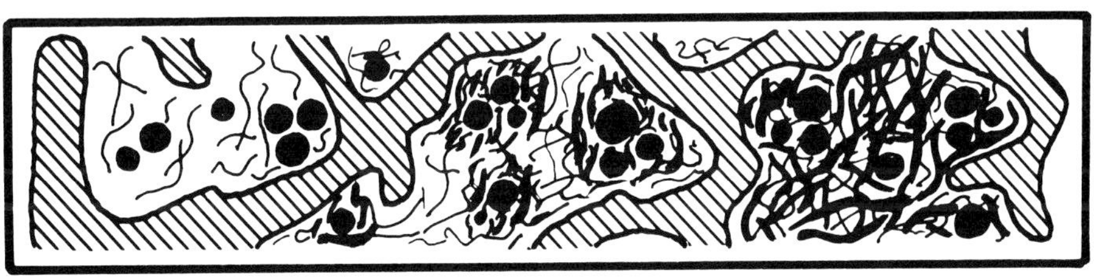

GRADE I GRADE II GRADE III

Figure 1 Degree of fibrosis in the bone marrow. Grade I: A diffuse increase in reticular fibers in the marrow parenchyme. Grade II: Both fine and coarse fibrosis around megakaryocytes and vessels. Grade III: Widespread coarse fibrosis.

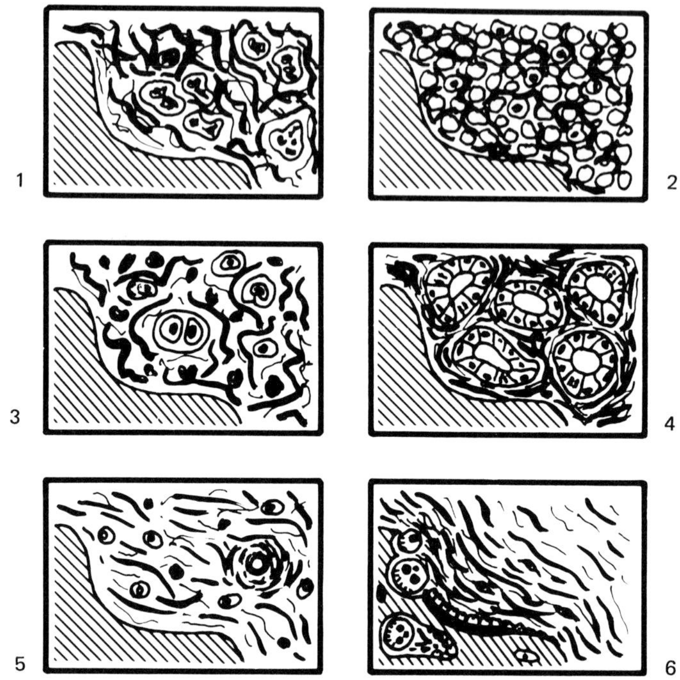

Figure 2 Underlying disorders and bone marrow fibrosis: 1. Myeloproliferative disorder; 2. lymphoproliferative disorder; 3. Hodgkin's disease; 4. carcinoma; 5. inflammatory; 6. hyperparathyroidism.

are given in Table 3. In all cases, complete replacement of hematopoietic tissue may eventually ensue.

Myelofibrosis (MF) and Osteomyelosclerosis (OMS) in the Myeloproliferative Disorders

Fibrosis in the bone marrow is initiated in association with specific structures and, in many cases, accompanied by certain features, and both are schematically represented in Figure 6.

The presence or absence of woven bone and/or appositional new bone in the biopsy was used for division of the patients into the two groups: those with MF or with OMS. The major clinical features are listed in Table 4, and the histologic and cytologic characteristics in Table 5. Megakaryocytes figured prominently in the development of both MF and OMS; their morpho-

Table 1 Bone Marrow Fibrosis[a] and Its Basic Disorders

Basic Disorders	Number of Patients
Hematologic neoplasias	
myeloproliferative disorders (MPD)	1255
acute/subacute leukemias (AL, SAL)	80
multiple myeloma (MM)	250
non-Hodgkin's lymphoma (NHL)	797
Hodgkin's disease (HD)	69
miscellaneous	78
Metastatic cancer	
breast	156
prostate	51
lung	32
others	27
unknown primaries	90
Inflammatory reactions	
toxic	38
infectious	8
unknown	42
Osteopathies	
Paget's disease	102
hyperparathyroidism (HPT)	112
Myelodysplasia	43
Total	3230

[a]Coarse fibrosis (grade II/III).

logic range is illustrated in Figure 7 and the frequency of the various types of megakaryocytes in the myeloproliferative disorders is given in Table 6.

Myelofibrosis/sclerosis developed particularly in those cases associated with proliferation of megakaryocytes. However, transition to a different myeloproliferative disorder also takes place in MF/OMS, and the frequency of its occurrence in our material was 12%. When the findings in the initial bone marrow biopsies were correlated with the patients' survival times, significant

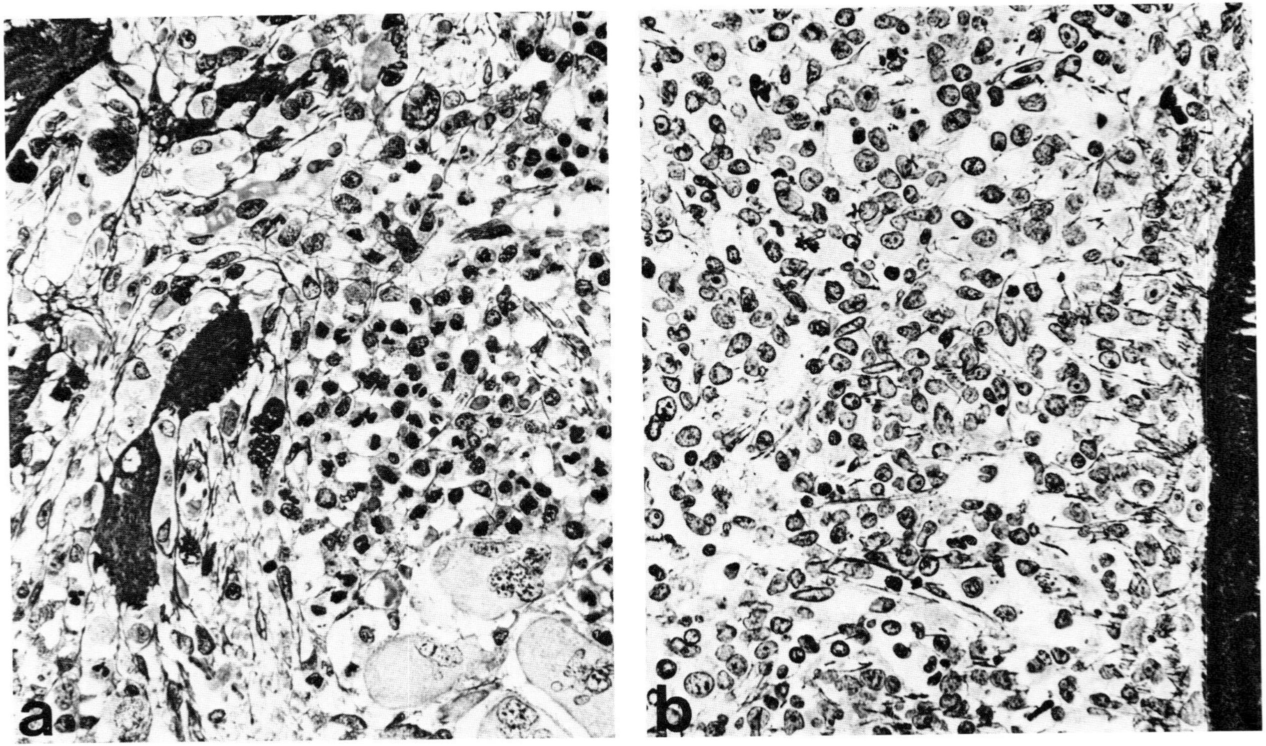

Figure 3 Patterns and etiologies of bone marrow fibrosis. Gomori stain, 250X. a. Myeloproliferative disorder; b. acute leukemia; c. non-Hodgkin's lymphoma; d. Hodgkin's disease; e. mammary carcinoma; f. Hand-Schüller-Christian disease; g. inflammatory, of unknown etiology; h. hyperparathyroidism.

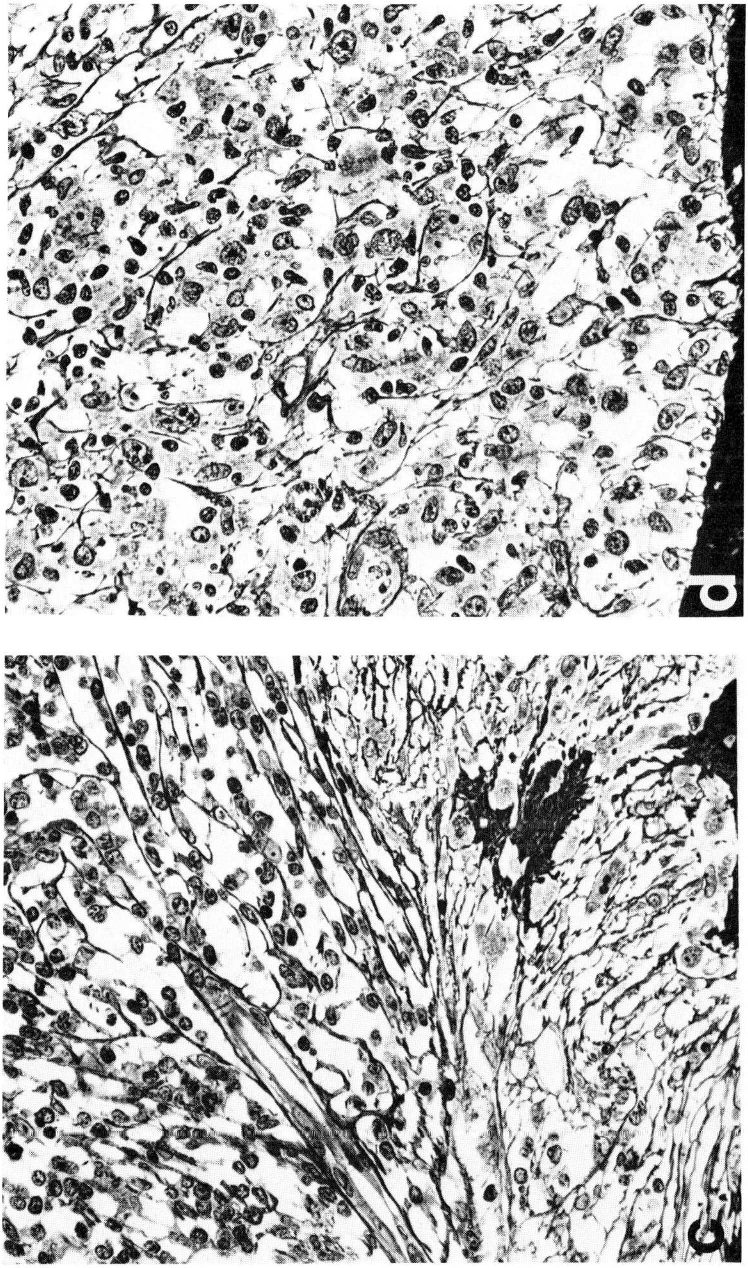

Figure 3 (continued).

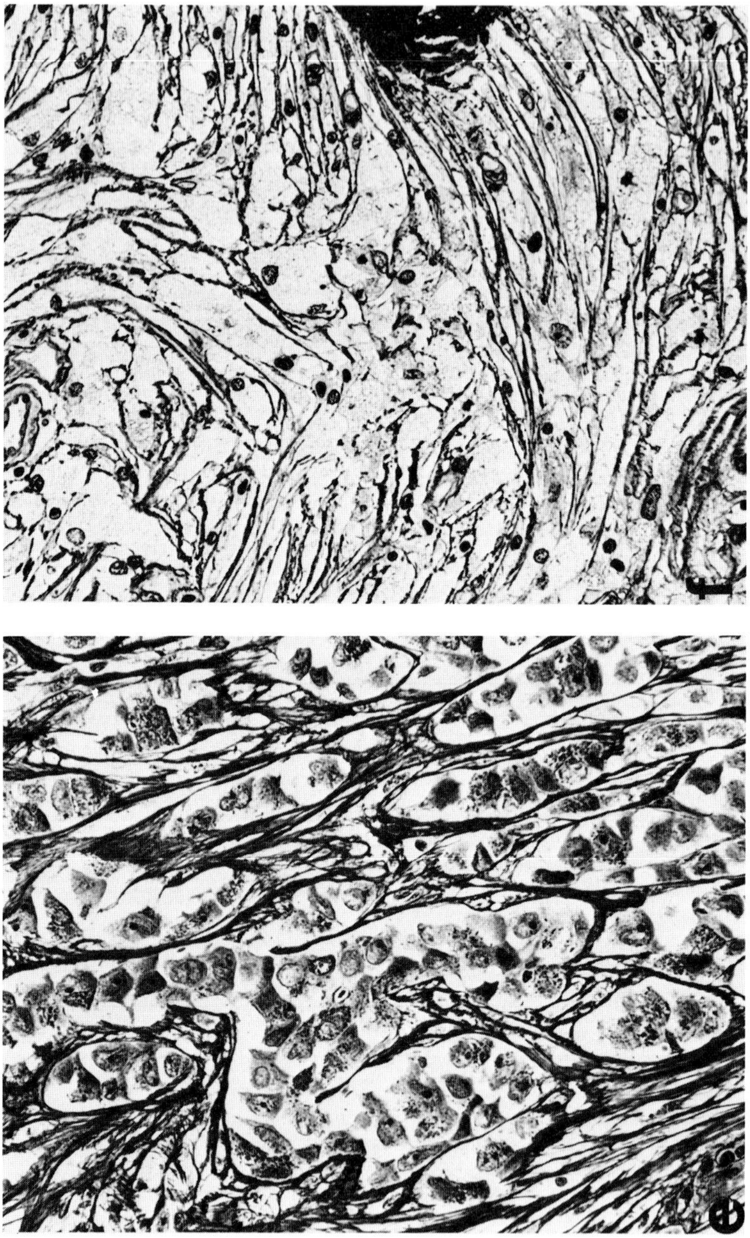

Figure 3 (continued).

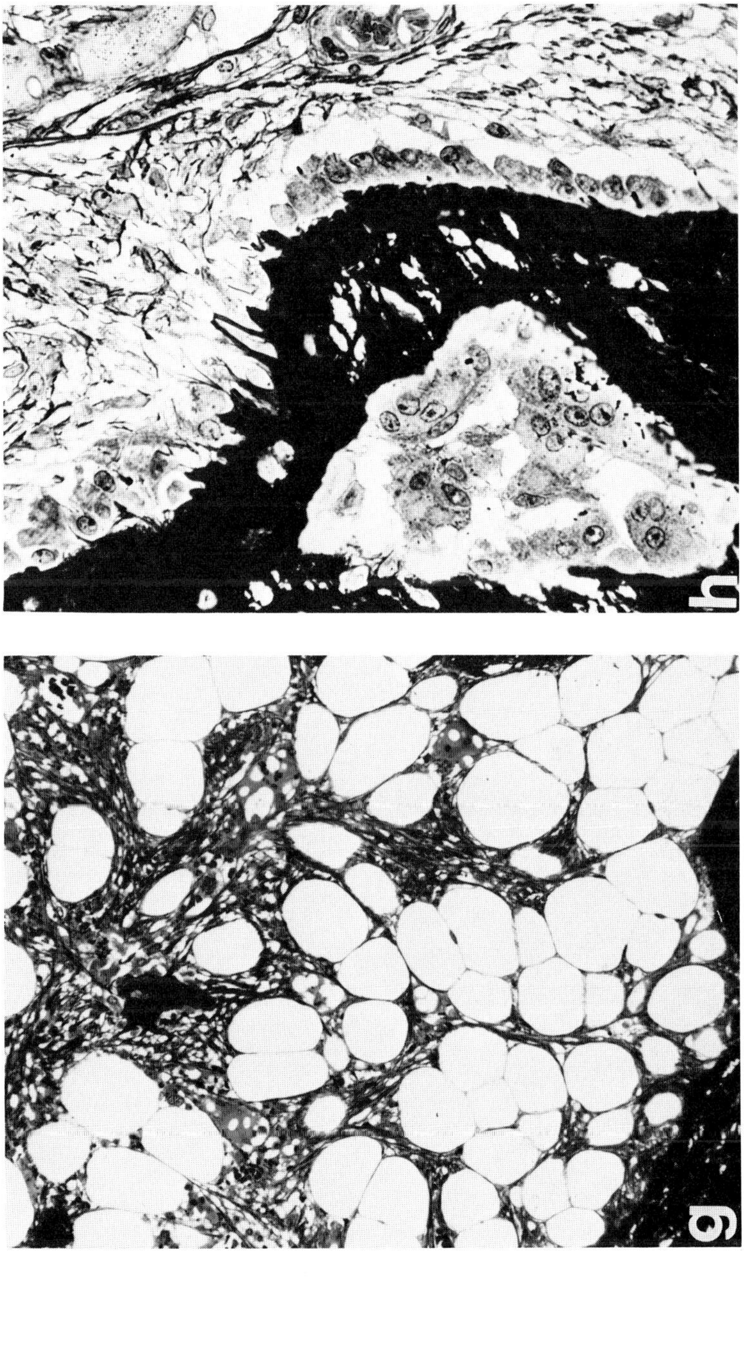

Figure 3 (continued).

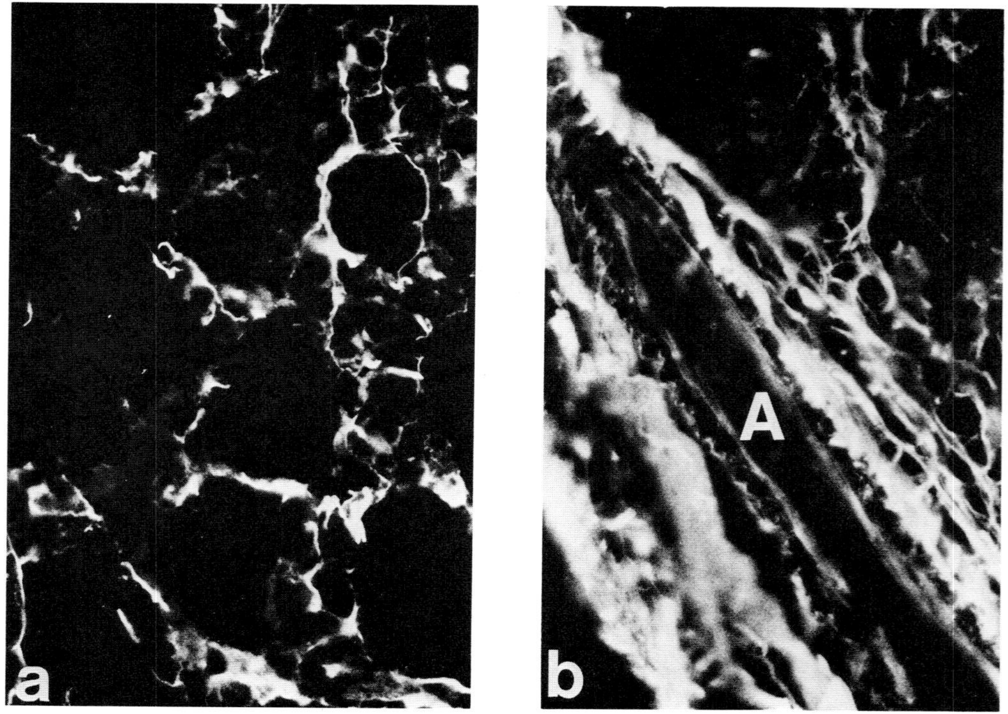

Figure 4 Collagen typing on fresh frozen sections of bone marrow (FITC): (a) type III, normal fiber pattern, 400X; (b) type III, normal perivascular fibers; A = lumen of an artery, 400X; (c) type I, layer of lamellar bone (l) as well as woven bone (W) within the marrow space both consisting of type I, 250X; (d) type III, collagen in endosteal mast cell granuloma, 250X.

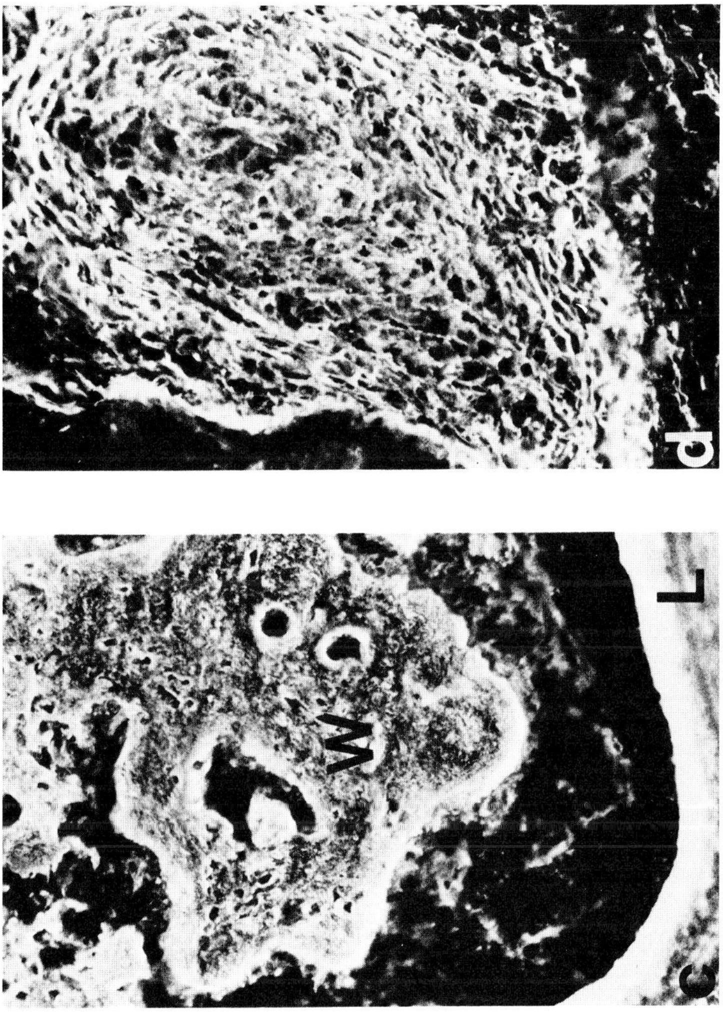

Figure 4 (continued).

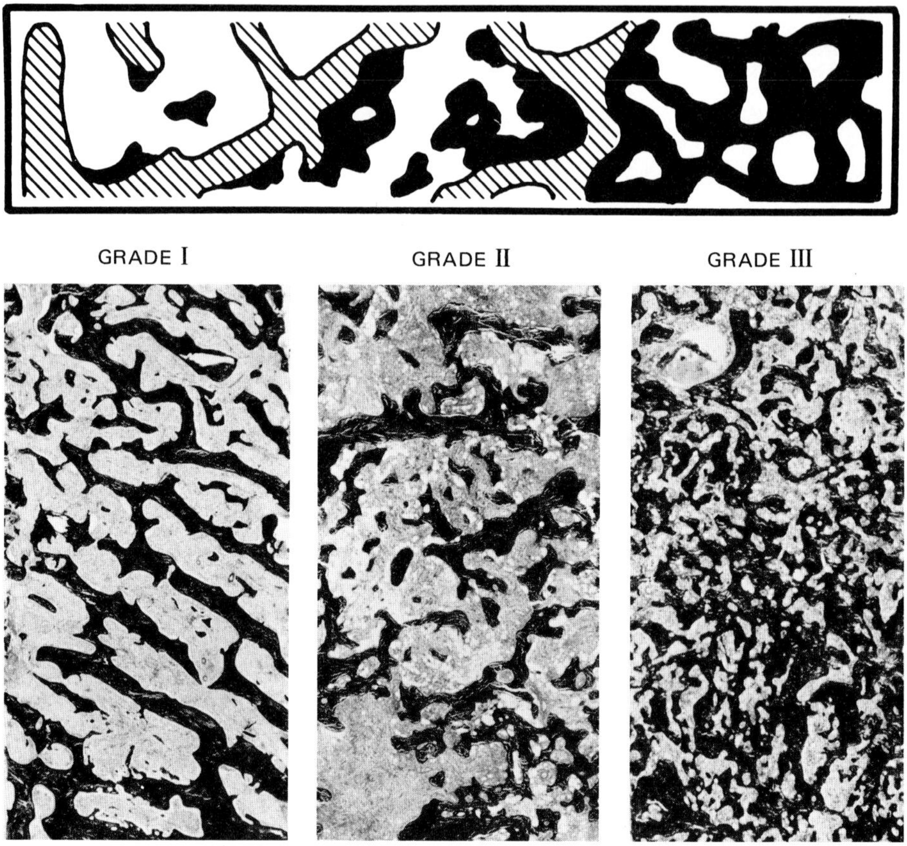

Figure 5 Degree of osteomyelosclerosis in the bone marrow. Gomori stain, 10X. Grade I: Small foci of primitive bone and increased trabecular appositional bone. Grade II: Increased appositional and woven bone in approximately equal proportions. Grade III: Almost complete replacement of normal trabecular architecture by a network of primitive bone.

Table 2 "Rapidly Progressive Bone Marrow Fibrosis"[a] and Its Basic Disorders

Basic Disorders[b]	Number of Patients
CML	8
MegM	7
PV	1
AL	12
SAL	8
MM	6
NHL	3
HD	2
Miscellaneous	6
Unknown	7
Total	60

[a]Histologic evidence of coarse fibrosis within 6 months of diagnosis.
[b]CML = Chronic myeloid leukemia; Meg M = megakaryocytic myclosis; PV = polycythemia vera. Other abbreviations are explained in Table 1.

differences were observed in certain disease groups, depending on type and degree of cellularity and the presence or absence of coarse fibrosis and/or woven bone (Table 7). Although some workers have also observed that an initially normo- or hypercellular bone marrow constitutes a favorable prognostic factor (5), others have not confirmed this (6).

Effect of Fibrosis on Hematopoiesis

Fibrosis in the bone marrow invariably resulted in the disruption of the normal architecture of the bone marrow, so that in many cases the hematopoietic precursors of the individual cell lines were segregated into separate areas (Fig. 8a) and frequently exhibited maturation arrest and other dysplastic features (Fig. 8b). The MPD are neoplastic proliferations, though capable (for varying periods of time) of producing differentiated progeny that are indistinguishable morphologically and functionally from their normal

Table 3 Fibrotic Patterns and Basic Disorders

Basic Disorders in the Bone Marrow[a]	Number of Patients	Normal Fibers (%)	Fibrosis Grade I (%)	Fibrosis Grade II (%)	Fibrosis Grade III (%)	Woven Bone (%)
		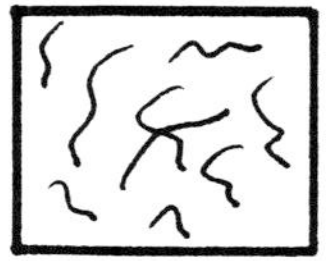	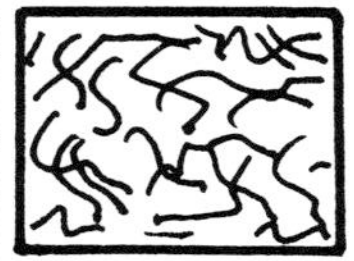	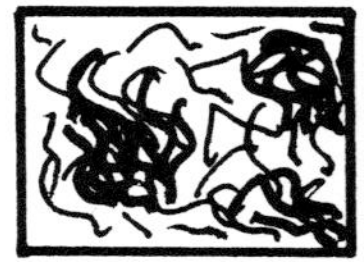	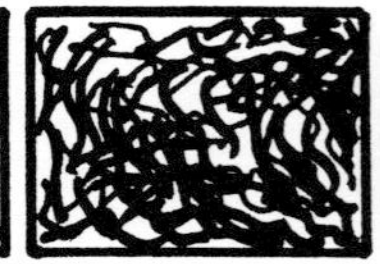	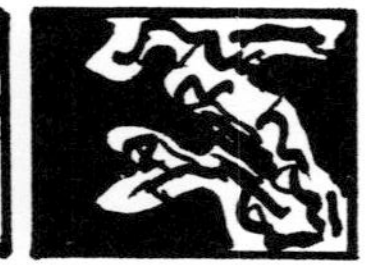
MPD	3393	28	35	11	14	12
AL	320	51	30	13	6	0
MM	813	32	37	20	9	2
NHL	1351	1	40	36	10	3
HD	95	0	27	30	39	4
Carcinoma	691	9	9	21	33	28
Sarcoma	60	2	20	28	30	20
HPT	280	15	45	20	16	9
Paget's disease	142	5	23	31	35	4

[a]For explanation of abbreviations, see Tables 1 and 2.

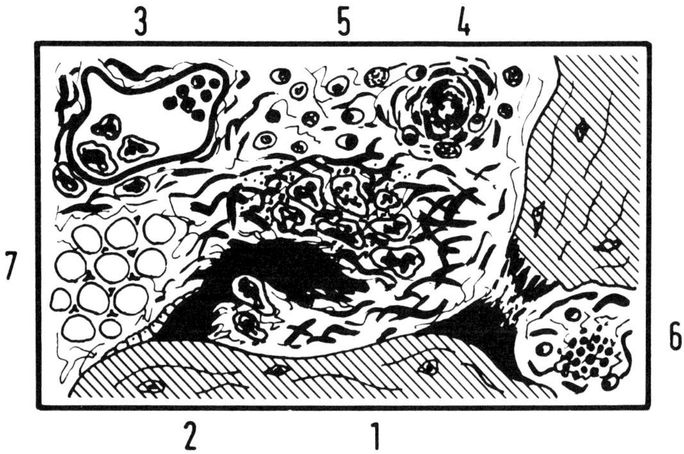

Figure 6 Histologic criteria in MF/OMS: (1 and 2) appositional and primitive bone formation; periosseous clusters of megakaryocytes and interstitial platelets. (3) Ectatic sinusoids with sclerotic walls and intravascular hematopoiesis. (4) Perivascular infiltration and fibrosis. (5) Inflammatory infiltrate of plasma, mast, and lymphoid cells. (6) Lymphoid cell aggregates. (7) Variable increase in fat cells.

counterparts. Residual normal hematopoiesis is present together with the malignant clone and both may show dysplastic maturation—the former because of its inherent abnormality and the latter because of alterations in the marrow architecture and therefore in the microenvironment in addition to the presence of the neoplastic clone (Fig. 8a, b). Of interest are the preservation of the fat cells (especially in OMS even in the presence of a reduction in hematopoietic tissue) and the differences in its distribution (Fig. 9)—paratrabecular in some cases and central intertrabecular in others.

It should be stressed that in the MPD the histology and the cytology of the bone marrow clearly reflect the stage of the disease at which the biopsy is taken: thus, in MF the marrow may typically be hypercellular with only incipient and developing fibrosis. The stimulation of the fibroblasts and fibers is accompanied by stromal (mesenchymal) activation including increased capillaries and blood flow. In many cases variable numbers of ectatic sinusoids are present, many containing hematopoietic precursors (Fig. 8a). There is also great variability in the number of iron-containing stromal cells and macrophages with crystalloid inclusions.

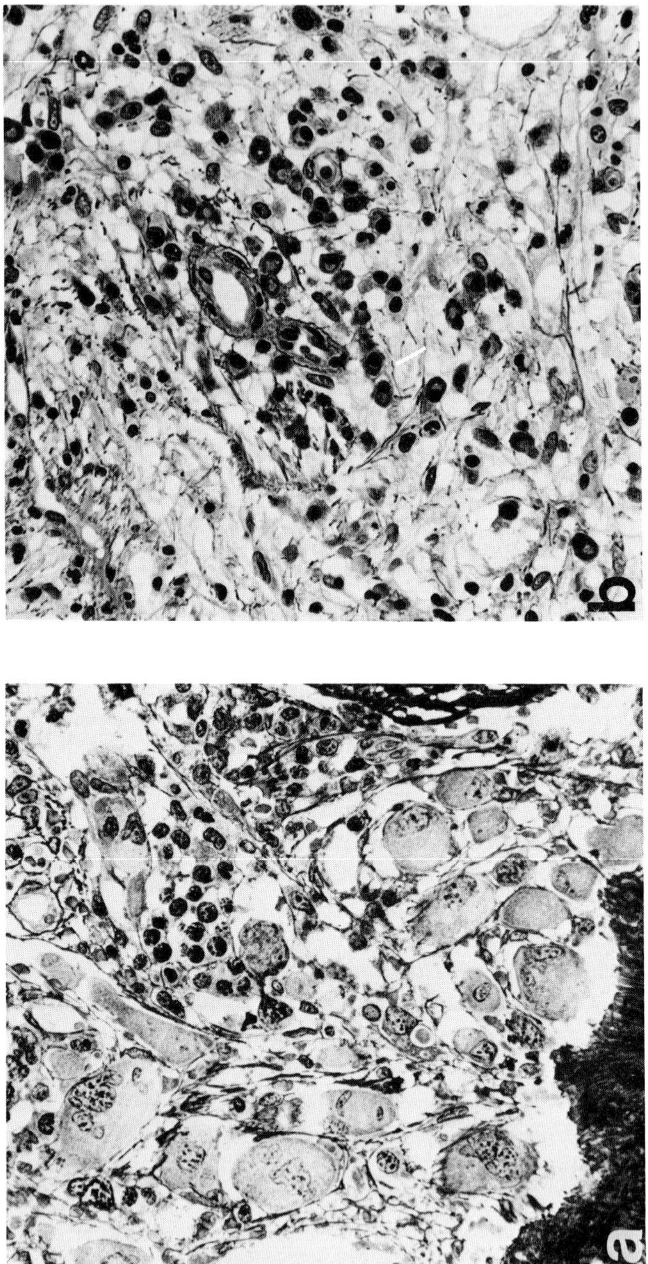
b
a

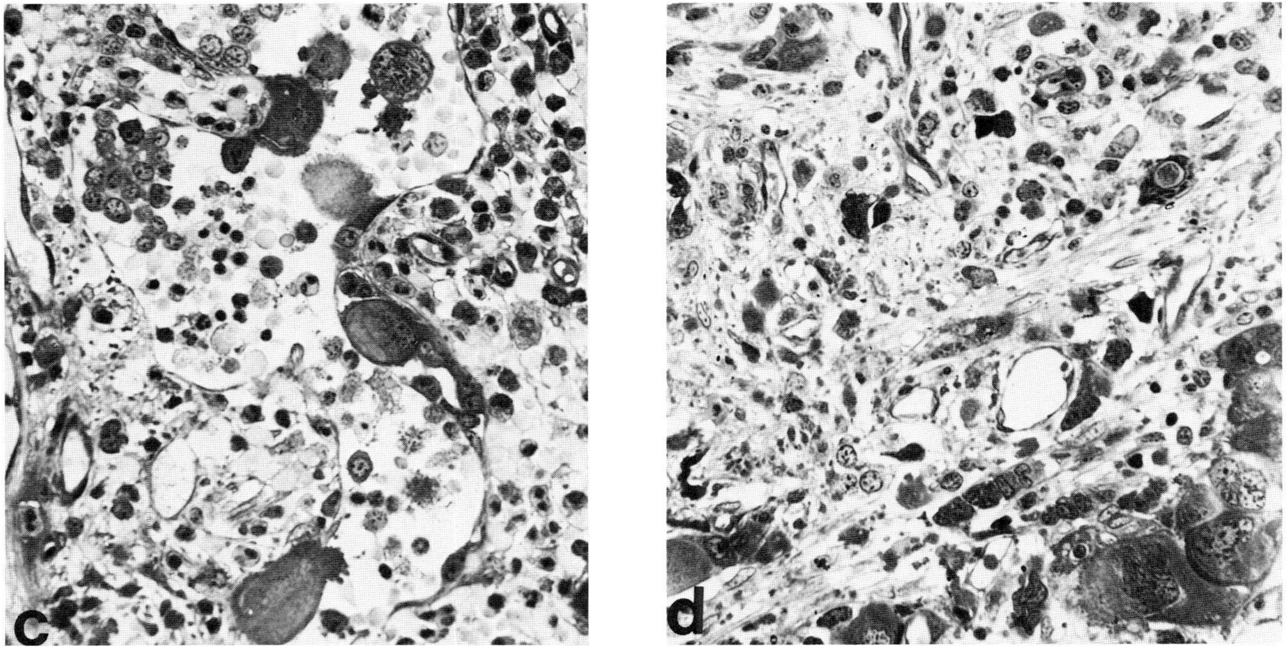

Figure 7 Cytologic characteristics in MF/OMS. (a) Cluster of megakaryocytes showing range in size and nuclear configuration; note fibers in their vicinity. Gomori stain, 400X. (b) Inflammatory infiltrate and edematous fibrotic marrow. Gomori stain, 400X. (c) Ectatic sinusoid with intraluminal erythroid and megakaryocyte precursors. Giemsa stain, 400X. (d) Megakaryocytes and platelets in interstitial space. Giemsa stain, 400X.

Table 4 Clinical Features of MF/OMs

	MF	OMS
Patients	607	437
Male/female	51/49	47/53
Age (years, median, range)	65 (17–88)	57 (10–81)
Symptom duration		
< 1 year	51%	44%
1–5 years	29%	33%
> 5 years	20%	23%
Hemoglobin < 10 g/dl	45%	35%
Hemoglobin > 16 g/dl	7%	3%
Leukocytes < 4×10^9/liter	16%	11%
Leukocytes > 10×10^9/liter	47%	47%
Platelets < 100×10^9/liter	34%	24%
Platelets > 400×10^9/liter	14%	13%
Peripheral normoblasts	27%	41%
Alkaline leukocyte phosphatase		
decreased	24%	37%
normal	21%	31%
increased	55%	32%
Dry tap	73%	70%
ESR, 2nd h	64	65
Iron (serum)		
decreased	50%	45%
normal	27%	37%
increased	23%	18%
Lactic dehydrogenose (serum), increased	81%	91%
Alkaline phosphatase (serum), increased	37%	50%
Splenomegaly	85%	94%
Hepatomegaly	71%	74%
Basic MPD		
polycythemia vera	18%	10%
idiopathic thrombocythemia	5%	4%
CML	20%	23%
unknown	49%	47%
Median survival (months)[a]	56	59

[a]From time of first biopsy to death or date of last contact.

Table 5 Histologic Characteristics of MF/OMS

	MF (n = 607)	OMS (n = 437)
Histomorphometry (vol%)		
hematopoiesis	46 (19)	20 (18)
fatty tissue	9 (9)	14 (14)
fibrous tissue	6 (8)	5 (4)
edema	7 (11)	6 (6)
sinusoids	8 (3)	7 (3)
trabecular bone	22 (8)	32 (14)
osteoid	2 (2)	6 (7)
woven bone	–	10 (17)
Osseous remodelling		
normal	82%	64%
osteoclastic	1%	4%
osteoblastic	12%	18%
osteoclastic/blastic	6%	14%
Trabecular bone volume		
decreased	51%	13%
normal	15%	2%
increased	12%	63%
irregular	22%	22%
Fibrosis		
grade I	4%	1%
grade II	39%	31%
grade III	57%	68%
Fatty tissue		
missing	41%	22%
decreased	47%	57%
normal	3%	5%
endostal increased	3%	3%
increased	6%	13%
Basic cell proliferation		
unclassifiable	5%	6%

Table 5 (Continued)

	MF (n = 607)	OMS (n = 437)
ERY/[a]	6%	6%
MEG/	16%	18%
PROMEG/	47%	51%
GRA	10%	9%
GRA/MEG	17%	11%
Siderin		
missing	11%	9%
decreased	27%	30%
normal	40%	38%
increased	22%	24%
Lymphoid nodules	23%	11%

[a]Basic cell proliferation ERY = erythrocytic; MEG = megakaryocytic; PROMEG = promegakaryocytic; GRA = granulocytic; GRA/MEG = granulocytic/megakaryocytic.

Prominent also in MF/OMS is the frequent occurrence of signs of an inflammatory reaction, in the form of zones of edema with eosinophils and mast cells, lymphocytes, and plasma cells (Fig. 7b). The significance of the single or multiple lymphoid cell aggregates found in about 15% of bone biopsies of patients with MPD, needs further clarification.

Pathogenesis of Fibrosis: Histologic Aspects

Various lines of evidence have now made it abundantly clear that fibrosis in the bone marrow is a secondary, reactive phenomenon (7–12). Its etiologies are manifold, and the fibrosis manifests itself to a variable extent in the different conditions. Though particular processes have been implicated in certain specific entities (13), there is most probably an interplay of causes in the majority of cases. For example, ineffective megakaryopoiesis with shedding of platelets and disintegration of megakaryocytes in the interstitium is thought to lead to release of megakaryocyte and platelet-derived growth factors (PDGF) and platelet factor 4 (PF4, an inhibitor of collagenase), which together bring about an increase in fibroblasts and fibers (9, 14). These functional studies have provided evidence to support earlier speculations on the role of megakaryocytes in myelofibrosis (8, 15, 16). The megakaryocyte compartment may be involved in the proliferation from the outset (17), or when

Table 6 Megakaryocytes in MPD

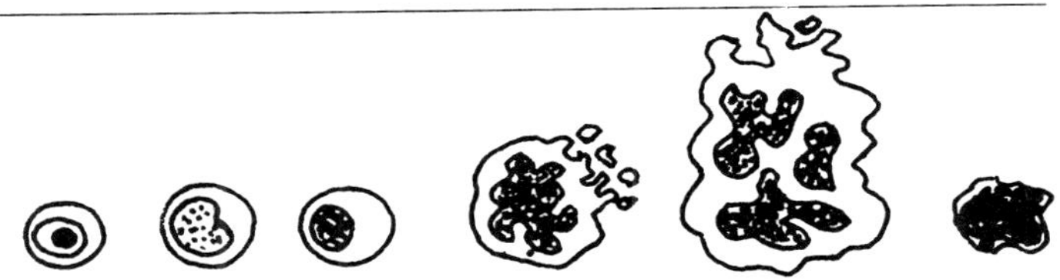

Proliferative Cell Series	Biopsies Number	Megakaryocytes[a]	1	2	3	4	5	6
ERY	22	810 (408)				+		+
ERY/GRA	34	876 (382)				+		+
ERY/MEG	104	6022 (4233)			+	++	+++	++
ERY/GRA/MEG	135	6820 (8210)			+	++	+++	++
MEG	77	19810 (20139)		+	++	++	+++	+++
GRA/MEG	97	8987 (6737)		+	++	+	+	
GRA		786 (520)		+	+			
PROMEG	68	31345 (22891)	+	+++	++			++
MEGBLAST	41	41710 (20312)	+++	+				++

[a]Mean (S.D.) of megakaryocytes per 100 mm^2 bone marrow area. 1 = megakaryoblast, 2 = promegakaryocyte, 3 = micromegakaryocyte, 4 = normal megakaryocyte, 5 = giant megakaryocyte, 6 = pyknotic megakaryocyte. Abbreviations are defined in Table 5.

Table 7 Predictive Value of Bone Marrow Fibrosis in Hematologic Malignancies

Clinical Entity[a]	Coarse Fibrosis[b]	Patients	Median Survival (Months)	Test Statistics (Mantel-Cox)[c]
PV	Absent	150	105	0.0002
	Present	125	61	
CML	Absent	162	24	0.0054
	Present	85	42	
AL	Absent	158	4	0.1243
	Present	20	2	
MM	Absent	118	65	0.0006
	Present	39	15	
NHL	Absent	319	36	0.0003
	Present	50	11	
HD	Absent	20	4	0.0629
	Present	49	9	

[a]For explanation of abbreviations see Table 1.
[b]Fibrosis grade II, III, and/or woven bone.
[c]Underlining indicates significant difference with $p < 0.05$ (BMDP 1L).

transformation occurs, as in megakaryoblastic transformation in chronic myelogenous leukemia (CML) (18, 19). A mixed myelomonoblastic and megakaryoblastic transformation in essential thrombocythemia has also been observed (20).

In many cases, more megakaryocytes may be present than suspected since characterization with specific enzymic and other markers (21) is required for unequivocal identification of megakaryoblasts and early megakaryocyte precursors; as the authors point out "recognition by conventional microscopy has remained very difficult if not impossible based mainly on subjective morphologic criteria." However, this applies less to undecalcified plastic-embedded bone marrow than to decalcified paraffin-embedded tissues.

There is a direct connection between megakaryocyte size, DNA content, and maturity of the cytoplasm (22). It has been shown that ploidy and maturity are linked: 95% of platelet-shedding megakaryocytes are in the 16 to 32 N range (Fig. 10a). Moreover, a certain cytoplasmic mass is also required, as the demarcation membrane system provides a membrane reserve for platelet production (23). Hence, hyperplasia of immature megakaryocytes is associated with a low platelet count. The extreme morphologic range in size, shape, nuclear configuration, cytoplasmic granularity, and density (2, 19, 24, 25) are exaggerations of megakaryocytic features that are to some extent normally present and that may also occur under conditions of stress due to increased demands as in hypersplenism, in thrombocytosis due to nonhematologic malignancies, or in preleukemic conditions as in the myelodysplastic syndromes (26). In MF/OMS (in the MPD), these megakaryocytic characteristics are undoubtedly an expression of dysplastic development due to their neoplastic transformation.

The ultimate fate of megakaryocytes in the human bone marrow is still unclarified: one mechanism may be release into the blood stream, as "naked" pyknotic megakaryocyte nuclei are frequently encountered in the sinusoids of the bone marrow. Another mechanism is phagocytosis by bone marrow macrophages, but so far this has been described in mice only (27). A third possibility is disintegration within the marrow interstitium, and when this is pathologically increased it results in augmented fibrosis, as in myeloproliferative disorders with megakaryocytic hyperplasia (Fig. 10b, c). Additional support has been adduced by study of megakaryocytes in the "gray platelet syndrome" (28) in which release of polypeptides from immature granules into the distended membrane system of megakaryocytes and hence to the outside, is associated with deficiency of granules in platelets, fibrosis in the bone marrow, and normal or high levels of PDGF and PF4 in plasma.

Etiologies and Contributing Factors: Histologic Correlations

The relatively frequent occurrence of lymphocytic infiltrates and lymphoid cell aggregates in the bone marrow in MPD has only recently been appreciated (29, 30); their presence may influence both fibrosis and hematopoiesis. The possible connection between them and the concomitant development of both a myelo- and a lymphoproliferative disorder has not yet been elucidated (31, 32).

Inflammatory mechanisms and activation of the complement system may also participate in fibrosis—as indeed may other specific factors either by their presence or by a relative deficiency.

The role of mast cells and the possible release of histamine and related substances must be considered when evaluating the inflammatory reactions in myelofibrosis; especially the edema and the increase in blood vessels, although angiogenic factors may be produced by other cells as well. When fibrosis follows inflammatory reactions, it is analogous to that occurring in

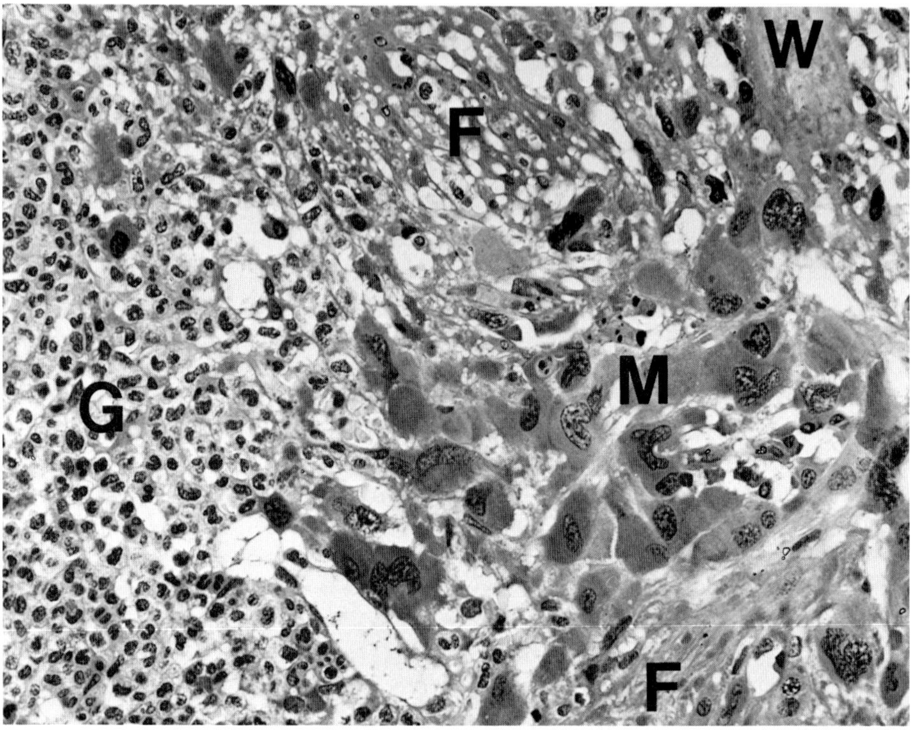

(a)

Figure 8 (a) Hypercellular phase of OMS; note woven bone (W), area of granulopoiesis (G) without fibrosis, and clusters of megakaryocytes (M) surrounded by coarse fibers (F). Giemsa stain, 400X. (b) Hematopoiesis in MF with marked dysplastic features; note dyserythropoiesis (D) megakaryocyte with multiple nuclei and micromegakaryocyte (M). Giemsa stain, 600X.

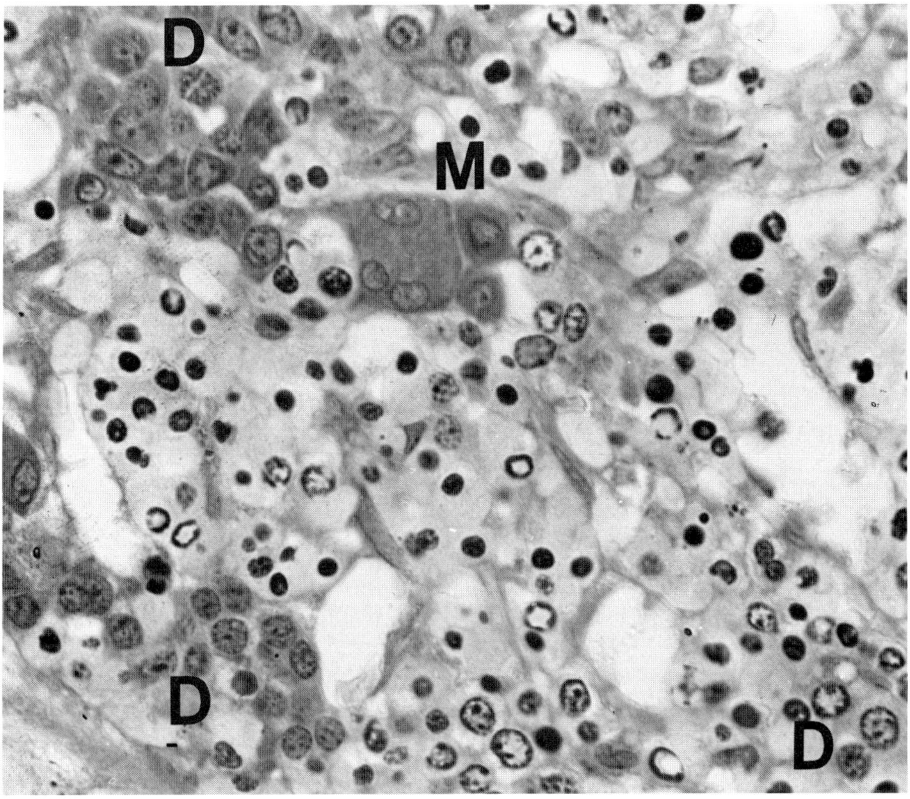

(b)

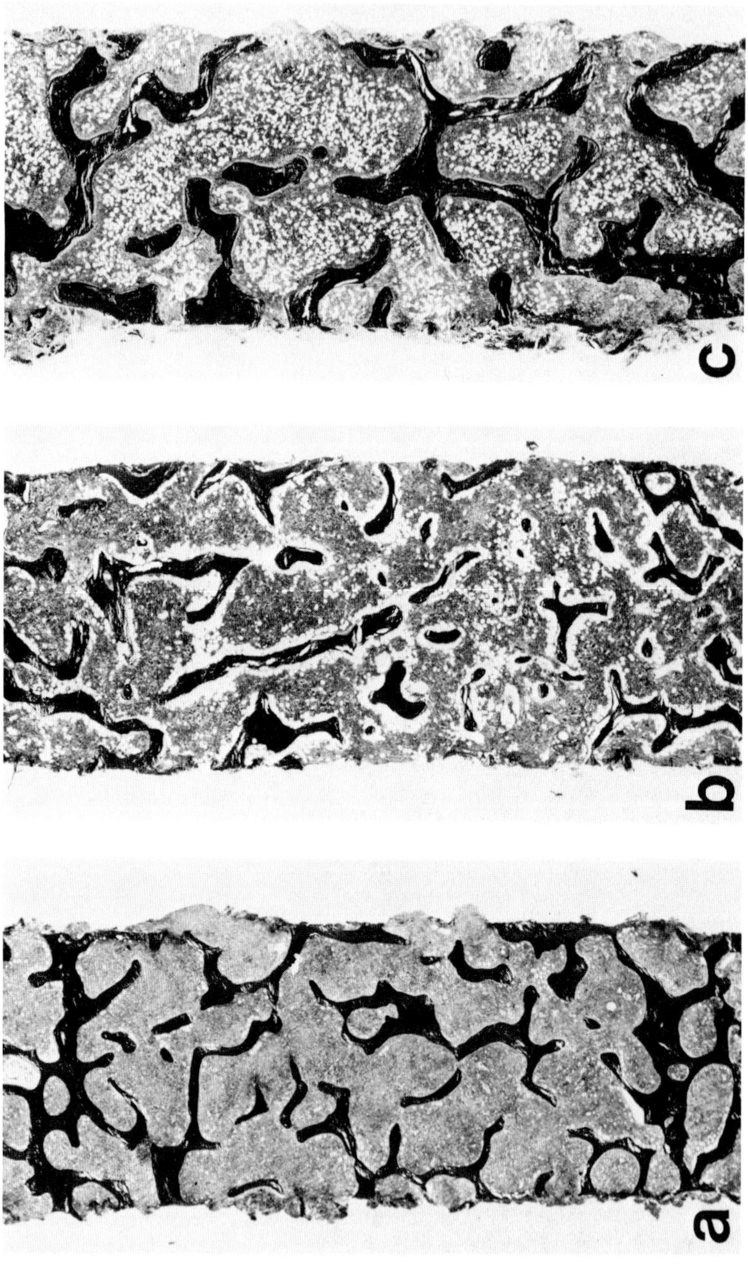

Figure 9 Histotopography of myelofibrosis. Gomori stain, 10X: (a) complete replacement of hematopoiesis by fibrosis; (b) intertrabecular fibrosis with paratrabecular preservation of fat cells; (c) paratrabecular fibrosis with increased fat within the marrow spaces.

other organs. The fibrosis accompanying these reactions is variable; in granulomatous disease fibers may be present in and around the granulomas, without an increase in the rest of the marrow (33, 34). The situation is more complicated when extramedullary neoplasias expand in the bone marrow. First, the normal tissues are replaced; second, these neoplasias consist of parenchyme (that is the tumor cells themselves) and connective tissue and blood vessels evoked by tumor cell factors and provided by the stromal tissues of the marrow (35, 36). In the bone marrow, the relative amounts of these two components vary greatly, from minimal stroma to an overwhelming fibrosis in which few tumor cells are identifiable (19, 37). Lymphomatous involvement of the bone marrow is almost always associated with some degree of fibrosis (32); mostly within the affected areas—a classic example is hairy cell leukemia—in some cases outside them as well, as in centrocytic lymphomas. In the latter, a pronounced osteoblastic reaction may also occur. Increased osseous remodeling due to factors (lymphokines) released by the tumor cells may accompany any malignant lymphoma in the bone marrow (38). Although both formation and resorption are generally affected, it may be primarily osteoblastic or osteolytic as in multiple myeloma, in which secretion of an osteoclast activating factor (OAF) is responsible. However, raised calcitriol levels in patients with lymphomas may also be associated with hypercalcemia (39).

It should be remembered that the skeleton constitutes a rigid bony cage with a fixed volume at any given time. When there is a decrease in hematopoietic tissue due to degeneration and necrosis, granulation tissue develops to take its place (as in healing processes elsewhere), but without the possibility of subsequent contraction to a smaller volume unless replacement by blood vessels, fat cells, or hematopoietic tissue ensues. Thus, fibrosis may follow necrosis as a result of nonspecific inflammatory processes or in the course of a myeloproliferative disorder, a lymphoproliferative disorder, in metastatic invasion of the bone marrow, after intensive chemotherapy, etc. (40).

In contrast, the connective tissue elements in diseases of bone can be considered an integral part of these disorders, as they accompany and are inseparable from the osseous manifestations: all are components of the mesenchyme, reacting to endocrine and other stimuli, notably parathyroid hormone, and vitamin D (41). It is now well established that 1,25-dihydroxyvitamin D, [1,25-(OH_2) D_3] the active metabolite of vitamin D, influences differentation of monocyte/macrophage precursors (preosteoclasts) (42) and thereby bone resorption (12, 43). However, it also has a role in bone formation and in the healing of rickets (12, 44). Recent studies have demonstrated that it inhibits megakaryocytic proliferation in culture (12) and that adminis-

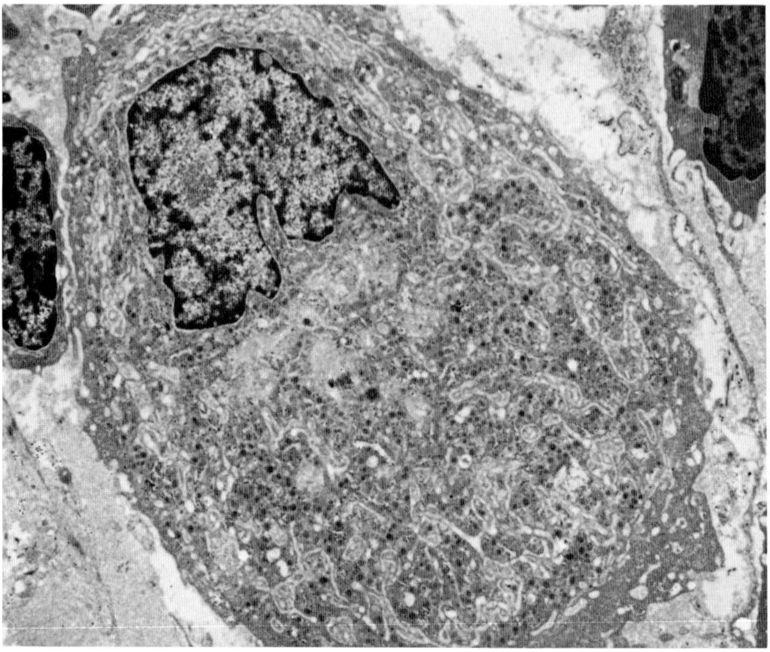

(a)

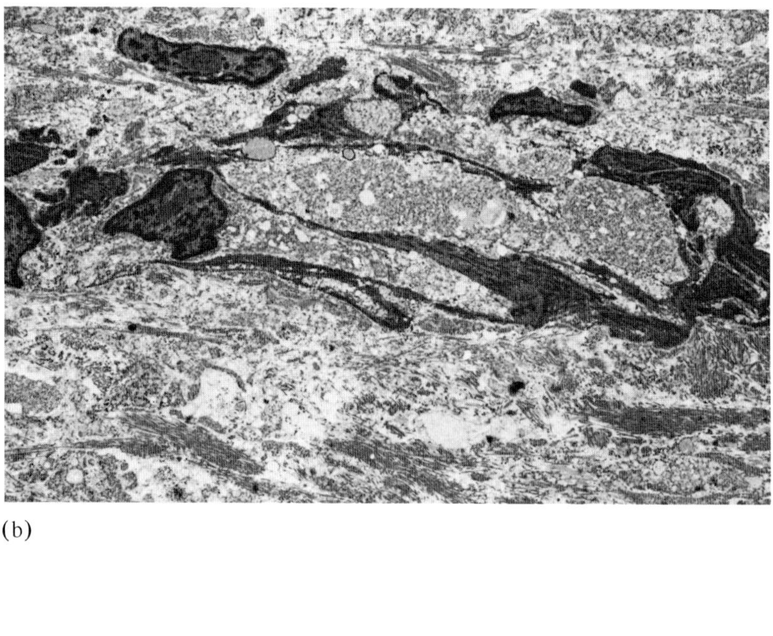

(b)

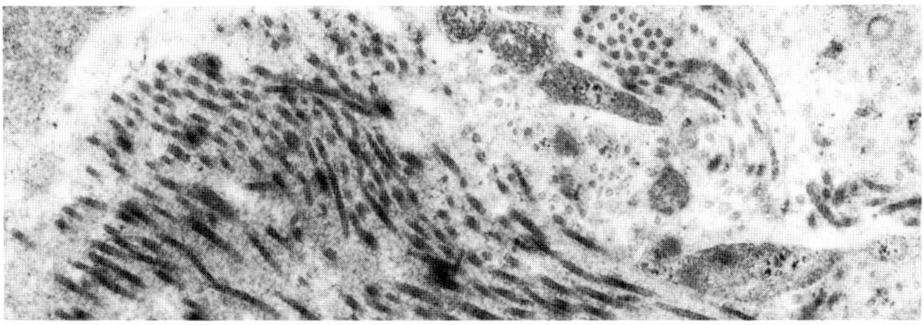

(c)

Figure 10 (a) EM of normal megakaryocyte; note membrane system demarcating platelets. 3200X. (b) Low-power view of bone marrow in myelofibrosis; note dysplastic megakaryocyte at right. 1600X. (c) High magnification of fibrotic area to show collagen fibers cut lengthways and in cross section. 16,000X.

tration of 1,25-(OH_2) vitamin D will reduce fibrosis in the bone marrow in some myeloproliferative disorders (45).

Histologic Variability and Stage of Disease

The variability of histology and cytology of the bone marrow in MF/OMS is due to the fact that it may be evoked at different stages of disease progression. Thus, there is a considerable range from acute myelofibrosis (46) in association with an acute megakaryoblastic, myeloblastic (or mixed) myelosis (17, 47–49) to an accelerated fibrosis accompanying a blastic crisis; a rapidly progressive fibrosis supervening in a chronic MPD; and finally the obliterative fibrosis occurring as a terminal phase in a chronic MPD (50). Consequently, in evaluating bone marrow histology and cytology, one must take into account both the underlying neoplastic MPD and the transitions it may undergo as part of its natural history. Therefore, variations in bone marrow histology and cytology in biopsies of individual patients, inevitably taken at different times of their disease, cannot be compared without taking these aspects into account, and it would be more useful to regard them as transitional phases in a wide spectrum within the MPD, rather than as presenting distinct and separable disease pictures. These considerations also apply when evaluating individual histologic characteristics as prognostic factors. Some investigations (6) have noted a marked variability in clinical severity and survival in "idiopathic" myelofibrosis, and these authors state that the degree of fibrosis and cellularity in bone marrow biopsies was of no prognostic significance, and a poor prognosis is related to "some unexplained primary marrow defect." Our observations indicate that the bone marrow histology, cytology, and degree of fibrosis do have prognostic significance, and the defect lies in the hematopoietic cells.

An intriguing question is raised by the presence of relatively large amounts of fatty tissue (rare in MF but not in OMS) and the lack of compensatory hematopoiesis in spite of the reduction in total active marrow space. In other situations (hemolysis, hypersplenism, leukemoid reactions) when a compensatory increase in hematopoiesis is required, fat cells are reduced. One can only speculate that the reason lies in the basically abnormal nature of the hematopoietic tissue (since it is a neoplastic clone) and in the altered microenvironment.

Hematopoietic Microenvironment and Fibrosis

An intact microenvironment is a prerequisite for the formation of "niches" for stem cells to settle in, for providing the cellular combinations required for directing differentiation to one or other cell line, for ensuring unperturbed and progressive maturation, and finally to enable unhindered egress from the marrow into the circulation. Even a small increase in connective tissue and fibers interferes with the bone marrow architecture and therefore with the microenvironment and thus contributes to many of the histologic, cytologic, and other characteristics of myelofibrosis–increase in circulating stem cells (51), compartmentalization of developing hematopoietic cell lines with dysplastic maturation and even degeneration and necrosis, sclerosis of vessels walls, and intravascular hematopoiesis. Recent studies have shown that bone marrow endothelial cells–an essential component of the marrow microenvironment–exercise a modulating influence on stem cells and on committed precursors (52). The disposition of the bone marrow sinusoids is profoundly disturbed, and their number is reduced in MF/OMS; this may be one reason for the compartmentalization of single cell lines observed in these conditions.

Unbalanced Mesenchymal Stimulation

Other questions are posed by the relationship—or lack of it—between fibroblast and osteoclast stimulation. It is of note that excessive osteoblastic bone formation is not seen in the presence of greatly increased fiber production [though recently a case of osteosclerosis occurring together with acute myelofibrosis has been reported (53)]. Possibly the production and diffusion of bone morphogenic factor (BMP) required for differentiation of osteoblasts (54) is hindered under these conditions so that an adequate local concentration is not reached. Moreover, osteoblastic bone formation and osteoclastic bone resorption in the adult organism are coupled and balanced processes, so that an increase or decrease in the one should lead to compensatory alterations in the other (55). Why there should be such an inadequate osteoclastic response to the augmented osteoblastic bone formation in OMS is completely unknown.

In the MPD, attenuation of trabeculae occurs in the absence of pronounced osteoclastic remodeling (56). In some cases, chronic hematopoietic hyperplasia is associated with accelerated bone turnover (57). However, osteolytic lesions have also been observed during the course of the disease and when a blastic crisis develops, possibly due to factors released by the neoplastic myeloid cells (58-61).

In some cases of OMS, there are thick seams of unmineralized osteoid, in others all the osteoid formed is calcified rapidly. When osteoclasts are present, they are more frequently observed on calcified bone to which they are attracted by chemotaxis, although they are capable of resorbing osteoid also as may be seen in osteomalacia and hyperparathyroidism. In OMS, clusters of megakaryocytes may be located at the trabecular bone surface; possibly these also interfere in some way with osteoclastic activity. Since osteoclasts are thought to be derived from a hematopoietic cell line (62, 63), altered hematopoiesis, perturbed marrow vasculature, and fibrosis impeding osteoclast migration to bone may be partially responsible. In addition, some tissue culture experiments have even implicated the vascular system in the origin of osteoclasts (64).

Histologic Diagnosis and Therapy

When painstaking anamnestic, physical, roentgenographic, biochemical, hematologic, and bone biopsy data are analyzed, most cases of idiopathic MF or agnogenic myeloid metaplasia will be found to have an identifiable cause (or at the very least, tentatively so). This is of considerable therapeutic importance because myelofibrosis is potentially reversible if the underlying cause may be treated. Lately, new avenues of approach have proved successful, especially in the myeloproliferative disorders. These treatments include cytotoxic therapy, splenectomy, bone marrow transplantation and administration of 1,25-(OH_2) vitamin D (44, 65-67).

ACKNOWLEDGMENT

The authors would like to express their gratitude to all colleagues who referred patients or sent biopsies. This work was supported by the Gesellschaft für Strahlen-und Umweltforschung mbH, Munich.

REFERENCES

1. Burkhardt, R. (1971). *Bone Marrow and Bone Tissue: Colour Atlas of Clinical Histopathology.* Berlin, Springer.
2. Bartl, R., Frisch, B., and Burkhardt, R. (1982). *Bone Marrow Biopsies Revisited. A New Dimension for Haematological Malignancies.* Basel, Karger.
3. Frisch, B., Bartl, R., and Burkhardt, R. (1982). Bone marrow biopsy in clinical medicine: an overview. *Haematologia 3*: 245–285.
4. Dixon, W. J., and Brown, M. B. (1979). *BMDP-79 Biomedical Computer Programs p-Series. System, Program and Statistical Development.* Berkeley, University of California Press.
5. Manoharan, A., Smart, R. C., and Pitney, W. R. (1982). Prognostic factors in myelofibrosis. *Pathology 14*: 445–461.
6. Varki, A., Lottenberg, R., Griffith, R., and Reinhard, E. (1983). The syndrome of idiopathic myelofibrosis. A clinicopathologic review with emphasis on the prognostic variables predicting survival. *Medicine 62*: 353–371.
7. Golde, D. W., Hocking, W. G., Quan, S. G., Sparkes, R. S., and Gale, R. P. (1980). Origin of human bone marrow fibroblasts. *Br. J. Haematol. 44*: 183–187.
8. Editorial anonymous. (1980). Myelofibrosis. *Lancet i*: 127–129.
9. Castro-Malaspina, H. and Moore, M. A. S. (1982). Pathophysiological mechanism operating in the development of myelofibrosis: Role of megakaryocytes. *Nouv. Rev. Fr. Hematol. 24*: 221–226.
10. Clare, N., Elsonk, D., and Manhoff, L. (1982). Cytogenic studies of peripheral myeloblasts and bone marrow fibroblasts in acute myelofibrosis. *Am. J. Clin. Pathol. 77*: 762–766.
11. Shah, I., Mayeda, K., Koppitch, F., Mahmood, S., and Nemitz, B. (1982). Karyotypic polymorphism in acute myelofibrosis. *Blood 60*: 841–
12. McCarthy, D. M., Hibbin, J., and Goldman, J. M. (1984). A role for 1,25-dihydroxyvitasmin D_3 in control of bone marrow collagen deposition? *Lancet i*: 78–80.
13. O'Donnell, J. R., Farrell, M. A., Fitzgerald, M. X., and O'Connell, L. G. (1982). Agnogenic myeloid metaplasia preceded by repeated leukemoid reactions and persistent acquired Pelger-Huet anomaly of granulocytes. Case report with review of acquired Pelger-Huet anomaly. *Cancer 50*: 1498–1505.
14. Berk, P., Malaspina, C., and Wasserman, L. (1983). Pathogenesis of myelofibrosis I: role of ineffective megakaryopoiesis and megakaryocyte components. New York, Grune & Stratton.
15. Hickling, R. A. (1937). Chronic non-leukaemic myelosis. *Q. J. Med. 6*: 253–275.

16. Burkhardt, R., Bartl, R., Beil, E., Demmler, K., Hoffmann, E., Irrgang, U., Kronseder, A., Langegger, H., Saar, U., Ulrich, M., and Wiemann, H. (1975). Myelofibrosis-osteomyelosclerosis syndrome–review of literature and histomorphology. *Adv. Biosci. 16*: 9–56.
17. Bevan, D., Rose, M., and Greaves, M., (1982). Leukaemia of platelet precursors: diverse features in four cases. *Br. J. Haematol. 51*: 147–164.
18. Williams, W. C., and Weiss, G. B. (1982). Megakaryoblastic transformation of chronic myelogenous leukaemia. *Cancer 49*: 821–926.
19. Frisch, B., Bartl, R., Burkhardt, R., Jäger, K., Mahl, G., and Kettner, G. (1984). Classification of myeloproliferative disorders by bone marrow histology. In *Bibl. haemat.*, No. 50. *Bone marrow biopsies updated. New prospects for clinical diagnosis.* Edited by B. Frisch, and R. Bartl. Basel, Karger, pp. 57–80.
20. Frei-Lahr, D., Barton, I. C., Hoffman, R., Burkett, L. L., and Prchal, J. T. (1984). Blastic transformation in essential thrombocythaemia. Dual expression of myelomonoblastic/megakaryoblastic phenotypes. *Blood 33*: 886–872.
21. Rabellino, E. M., Levene, R. B., Nachman, R. L., and Leung, L. L. K. (1984). Human megakaryocytes III. Characterization in myeloproliferative disorders. *Blood 63*: 615–622.
22. Levine, R. F., Hazzard, K. C., and Lamberg, J. D. (1982). The significance of megakaryocyte size. *Blood 60*: 1122–1131.
23. Radley, J. M., and Haller, C. J. (1982). The demarcation membrane system of the megakaryocyte: a misnomer? *Blood 60*: 213–219.
24. Georgii, A., Thiele, J., and Vykoupil, K. F. (1980). Osteomyelofibrosis/sclerosis: a histological and cytogenetic study on core biopsies of the bone marrow. *Virch. Arch. A. Pathol. Anat. Histol. 389*: 269–286.
25. Thiele, J., Holgado, S., Choritz, H., and Georgii, A. (1983). Density distribution and size of megakaryocytes in inflammatory reactions of the bone marrow (myelitis) and chronic myeloproliferative diseases. *Scand. J. Haematol. 31*: 329–341.
26. Wheeler, L. A., Hogan, R. P., Schwenk, G. C., and Griep, J. A. (1983). Multinucleate megakaryocytes in refractory anemia with excess blasts. *Arch. Pathol. Lab. Med. 107*: 277–278.
27. Radley, J. M., and Haller, C. J. (1983). Fate of senescent megakaryocytes in the bone marrow. *Br. J. Haematol. 53*: 227–287.
28. Deschamps, J. F., and Caen, J. P. (1984). Abnormal megakaryocyte release and myelofibrosis. *Lancet i*: 567–568.
29. Hernandez, N. L., Sureder, M. M., Granena, A., et al. (1979). Bone marrow lymphoid follicles in MF compared with CML. *Nouv. Rev. Franc. Hemat. 21*: 251–256.
30. Jäger, K., Burkhardt, R., Bartl, R., Frisch, B., and Mahl, G. (1983). Lymphoid infiltrates in chronic myeloproliferative disorders (MPD). *Verh. Dtsch. Ges. Path. 67*: 239–242.

31. Jennings, W., Chin-Yang, L., and Kiely, J. M. (1983). Concomitant myelofibrosis with agnogenic myeloid metaplasia and malignant lymphoma. *Mayo Clin. Proc. 58*: 617–619.
32. Bartl, R., Frisch, B., Burkhardt, R., Jäger, K., Pappenberger, R., and Hoffmann-Fezer, G. (1984). Lymphoproliferations in the bone marrow: identification and evolution, classification and staging. *J. Clin. Pathol. 37*: 233–254.
33. Bodem, C. R., Hamory, B. H., Taylor, H. M., and Kleopfer, L. (1983). Granulomatous bone marrow disease—a review of the literature and clinicopathologic analysis of 58 cases. *Medicine 62*: 372–383.
34. Schlag, R., Burkhardt, R., Bartl, R., and Kettner, G. (1983). Acute and chronic inflammatory changes in the bone marrow. *Verh. Dtsch. Ges. Path. 67*: 474–477.
35. Schor, A. M., and Schor, S. L. (1983). Tumour angiogenesis. *J. Pathol. 141*: 385–413.
36. Iozzo, R. V. (1984). Proteoglycans and neoplastic-mesenchymal cell interactions. *Human Pathol. 15*: 2–10.
37. Hernandez-Nieto, L., Muncunill, J., Rozman, C., Fabregues, M., Feliu, E., Granena, A., Montserrat-Costa, E., and Nomdedeu, B. (1978). Secondary myelofibrosis and/or osteosclerosios. An assessment of 400 biopsies. *Sangre 23*: 402–410.
38. Gowen, M., Wood, D. D., McGuire, M. K. B., and Russell, R. G. G. (1983/84). Stimulation of bone resorptilon in vitro by human interleukin 1. *Met. Bone Dis. Rel. Res.* V.S. No.
39. Breslau, N. A., McGuire, J. L., Zerwekh, J. E., Frenkel, E. P., and Pak, C. Y. C. (1984). Hypercalcemia associated with increased serum calcitriol levels in three patients with lymphoma. *Ann. Int. Med. 100*: 1–7.
40. Bain, B. (1980). Extensive bone marrow infarction followed by myelofibrosis in a patient with PH' positive chronic granulocytic leukaemia. *J. Clin. Pathol. 33*: 449–453.
41. Stavros, C. M., and Deftos, L. J. (1984). The vitamin D endocrine system and the hematolymphopoietic tissue. *Ann. Int. Med. 100*: 144–146.
42. Freake, H. C., McCarthy, D. M., San Miguel, J. F., Green, P. M., Zola, H., Catovsky, D., Goldman, J., and Macintyre, I. (1983/84). $1,25(OH)_2D_3$ Causes monocytic differentiation of normal human bone marrow in vitro. *Met. Bone Dis. Rel. Res.* V.S. No.
43. Editor anonymous. (1984). Vitamin D and the lymphomedullary system. *Lancet i*: 1105–1106.
44. Dickson, I. R., Hall, A. K., and Jande, S. S. (1983/84). DO $1,25(OH)_2$ vitamin D_3 and $24,25(\ /H)_2$ have a role in bone formation and in the healing of rickets? *Met. Bone Dis. Rel. Res.* V.S. No.
45. Arlet, P., Nicodeme, R., Adoue, D., Larregain-Fournier, D., Delsol, G., and Le Tallec. (1984). Clinical evidence for 1,25-Hydroxycholecalciferol action in myelofibrosis. *Lancet i*: 1013–1014.

46. Lewis, S. M., and Szur, L. (1963). Malignant myelosclerosis. *Br. Med. J. 2*: 472–477.
47. Strebel, U., Schaffner, A., and Fehr, J. (1983). Die akute Osteomyelofibrose. Eine Übersicht anhand von zwei eigenen Fällen. *Schweiz. Med. Wschr. 113*: 844–850.
48. Mahl, G., Frisch, B., Bartl, R., Burkhardt, R., Jäger, K. and Pappenberger, R. (1983). Acute myelofibrosis: Only one extreme of the spectrum of idiopathic myelofibrosis. *Verh. Dtsch. Ges. Path. 67*: 272–275.
49. Truong, L. D., Saleem, A., and Schwartz, M. R. (1984). Acute myelofibrosis. A report of four cases and review of the literature. *Medicine 63*: 182–187.
50. Bergsman, K. L., and van Slyck, E. J. (1971). Acute myelofibrosis. An accelerated variant of agnogenic myeloid metaplasia. *Ann. Int. Med. 74*: 232–235.
51. Wang, J. C., Cheung, C. P. Fakhiuddin, A., Steier, W., and Tobin, M. S. (1983). Circulating granulocyte and macrophage progenitor cells in primary and secondary myelofibrosis. *Br. J. Haematol. 54*: 301–307.
52. Ascensao, J. L., Vercellotti, G. M., Jacob, H. S., and Zanjani, E. D. (1984). Role of endothelial cells in human hemtopoiesis: modulation of mexid colony growth in vitro. *Blood 63*: 553–558.
53. Karasick, S., Karasick, D., and Schilling, J. (1982). Acute megakaryoblastic leukemia (acute malignant myelofibrosis): An unusual cause of osteosclerosis. *Skel. Radiol. 9*: 45–46.
54. Nogami, H., and Oohira, A. (1984). Postnatal new bone formation. *Clin. Orthop. Rel. Res. 184*: 106–113.
55. Rasmussen, H., and Bordier, P. (1974). The physiological and cellular basis of metabolic bone disease. In *Bone Cells–Morphology and Physiology*. Baltimore, Williams and Wilkins Co., chapter 2, pp. 8–70.
56. Burkhardt, R., Frisch, B., Bartl, R., Mahl, G., Jäger, K., Schlag, R., and Hill, W. (1984). Myelogenous osteodysplasia: Diagnosis and development. (Submitted for publication.)
57. Weinstein, R. S., and Lutcher, C. L. (1983). Chronic erythroid hyperplasia and accelerated bone turnover. Pergamon Press. *Metab. Bone Dis. Rel. Res. 5*: 7–12.
58. Habner, C. B. A., Haskill, C. M., and Canellos, G. P. (1969). Destructive bone lesions in chronic granulocytic leukemia. *Medicine (Baltimore) 48*: 401–410.
59. Mora, J. J., Heron, J. F. L'Hirondel, J. C., and Loyau, G. (1979). Lesion osteolytique au cours de la leucemie myeloid chronique. *Nouv. Presse. Méd. 8*: 3171.
60. Kosmidis, P. A., Palacos, C. G., and Axelrod, A. R. (1980). Diffuse purely osteolytic lesions in myelofibrosis. *Cancer 46*: 2263–2265.
61. Walther, R. M., and Greenberg, B. R. (1980). Hypercalcemia in the accelerated phase of chronic myelogenouos leukemia. *Cancer 46*: 1174–1178.

62. Chalmers, T. J. (1980). Cellular basis of bone resorption. *Clin. Orthop. Rel. Res. 151*: 283–293.
63. Owen, M. (1980). Origin of bone cells in the postnatal organism. *Arthritis Rheumat. 23*: 1073–1080.
64. Shimomuro, Y., and Suzuki, F. (1984). Cultured growth cartillage cells. *Clin. Orthop. Rel. Res. 184*: 93–105.
65. Clough, V., Geary, C. G., Hashmi, K., Davson, J., and Knowlson, T. (1979). Myelofibrosis in chronic granulocytic leukaemia. *Br. J. Haematol. 42*: 515–526.
66. Oblon, D. J., Elfenbein, G. J., Braylan, R. C., Jones, J., and Weiner, R. S. (1983). The reversal of myelofibrosis associated with chronic myelogenous leukemia after allogneic bone marrow transplantation. *Exp. Hematol. 4*: 681–685.
67. Richman, C. M., Rowley, J. D., and Golomb, H. M. (1984). Chronic granulocytic leukemia: epidemiology and etiology, pathogenesis, cytogenetics, in vitro studies and clinical features. In *Leukemias.* Edited by J. M. Goldman, and H. D. Preisler, London, Butterworths International Medical Reviews.

4

Biology and Pathobiology of Bone Marrow Connective Tissue

STUART A. BENTLEY
University of North Carolina, Chapel Hill, North Carolina

INTRODUCTION

Proliferation of connective tissue elements within the bone marrow is a constant feature in myelofibrosis, to the extent that the diagnosis is virtually insupportable in its absence. This finding is not, however, pathognomonic, as it occurs to a greater or lesser extent in association with a wide variety of bone marrow lesions, either as a local reaction or as a generalized process, involving the entire hematopoietic tissue. The class of diseases most consistently associated with marrow fibrosis is the myeloproliferative group and, within this group, fibrosis tends to be most prominent in myelofibrosis.

Myelofibrosis, characterized by the triad of marrow fibrosis, leukoerythroblastic anemia, and extramedullary hematopoiesis, was first described by Hueck (1) in 1879 (see also Chapter 1). Early investigators, aware of the association of marrow fibrosis with such disorders as tuberculosis and metastatic carcinomatosis, regarded fibrosis as the primary lesion, occurring in response to some unidentified agent. Anemia was thought to result from fibrotic infiltration of the marrow, with extramedullary hematopoiesis as a compensatory mechanism.

Certain features of myelofibrosis, however, are not explicable in terms of the latter model. The most important of these features is the association of the disorder with conditions characterized by excessive proliferation of bone marrow elements. Damashek (2) first proposed the inclusion of myelofibrosis in the same general classification as polycythemia vera, essential thrombocythemia, and chronic granulocytic leukemia, and first applied the term "myeloproliferative syndromes" to the group.

The original classification of myelofibrosis as a myeloproliferative disorder was based on the assumption that bone marrow connective tissue elements and hematopoietic elements share a common stem cell. The recent demonstration that hematopoietic elements in myelofibrosis are clonally derived justifies the inclusion of myelofibrosis within the myeloproliferative group, but these studies have also demonstrated that bone marrow fibroblasts are not derived from the neoplastic clone (3). Marrow fibrosis would thus appear to be a reaction to a stimulus emanating from hematopoietic cell proliferation and not, as suggested by Damashek, a primary neoplastic process involving marrow stromal elements. More recent evidence suggests that at least a subpopulation of marrow stromal elements may be derived from hematopoietic stem cells (4). The significance of marrow fibrosis in relation to the myeloproliferative disorders thus remains a controversial subject.

The etiology and pathogenesis of the myeloproliferative syndromes in general and of myelofibrosis in particular remain uncertain. A complete understanding of the biological relationship of marrow fibrosis to the underlying pathogenetic process therefore must await developments in these more fundamental areas.

Major advances have been made in recent years. New knowledge derived from a variety of disciplines, including collagen biochemistry and histochemistry, bone marrow ultrastructure, hematopoietic cell culture, and cell growth regulation, provides the potential for new initiatives in the investigation of myelofibrosis. Potentially relevant developments in these areas will now be reviewed and their significance with respect to the pathological processes underlying myelofibrosis will be discussed.

THE BIOCHEMISTRY OF COLLAGEN

A detailed analysis of collagen biochemistry is beyond the scope of this publication, and the discussion that follows represents only a brief summary of the relevant subject matter. For more complete coverage, the reader is referred to appropriate review articles, such as that of Bornstein and Traub (5).

Table 1 Genetically Distinct Collagens

Type	Molecular Chain Composition	Native Polymer	Tissue Distribution
I	Alpha 1(I)2 alpha 2(I)	Fibril	Skin, bone, tendon ligament, dentin, blood vessels, interstitial connective tissue
II	Alpha 1(II)3	Fibril	Cartilage, nucleus pulposus, vitreous body
III	Alpha 1(III)3	Fibril	As type I, except for bone and tendon; prominent in blood vessels
IV	Alpha 1(IV)/alpha 2(IV)	Network	Basement membranes
V	Alpha 1(V)2 alpha 2(V)	Unknown	Extensive: muscle, basement membranes, etc.

Collagens have been shown to be the product, not of a single gene, but of a family of closely related but structurally distinct genes. Collagens derived from separate genes are referred to as collagen types, of which five have so far been defined. The subunit structures and biological distributions of these collagen types are summarized in Table 1. Collagen types 1, 2, and 3 form extracellular fibers and are often referred to as "interstitial collagens." Collagen types 4 and 5 are found primarily in epithelial basement membranes.

The collagens as a group are defined on the basis of a characteristic quaternary structure, consisting of three polypeptide chains (alpha-chains) arranged in a triple helix. Although similar quaternary structure may be observed regionally within certain proteins that are generally regarded as noncollagenous, such as acetylcholinesterase and the complement component C1q, the triple helix is otherwise unique.

Collagen Structure

The helical domains of collagen alpha-chains consist of a repeating sequence of amino acid triplets of which glycine is invariably the first member. The structure may thus be represented as $(\text{Gly-X-Y})_n$, where X and Y may be any amino acid. The alpha-chains of interstitial collagens are usually about 1000 amino acid residues in length, with molecular weights in the region of 95,000-100,000. The factor n is thus about 333. Glycine is the major amino acid in the alpha-chain, comprising 33.3% of the molecule, whereas proline and hydroxyproline comprise about 20%. Hydroxyproline and hydroxylysine are found only in collagen.

The triple helical structure of collagen appears to be determined by the primary structure of the alpha-chains. A triple helix is assumed spontaneously by a variety of synthetic polypeptides. Polyglycine forms a highly stable and insoluble triple helix. Synthetic polypeptides consisting of amino acid triplets, analogous to collagen alpha-chains, exhibit variable tendencies to form triple helices. Thus, chains of the structure (Gly–Pro–Ala)$_n$ form helices spontaneously, whereas (Gly–Ala–Pro)$_n$ chains do not. The molecular basis for these observations is unclear.

The alpha-chain secondary structure is a left-handed helix with a periodicity of three residues per turn. The tertiary structure within the triple helix is a supercoil with a periodicity of approximately 39 residues per turn. Glycine residues within the triple helix are staggered by one residue. The final result is an elongated molecule approximately 300 nm in length and 5 nm in diameter.

Interstitial collagens form extracellular fibrillar aggregates in connective tissues. The basic subunit appears to a five-stranded microfibril with a cross-banded appearance in electron micrographs. This D-banding displays a periodicity of 68 nm and is due to staggering of collagen molecules within the microfibril.

Collagen Biosynthesis

Mapping of the chick collagen alpha 2(I) gene indicates that the chain is transcribed from at least 51 exons distributed over a 37-kb region. Transcription thus involves at least 51 distinct excision and splicing events. The role of the intervening sequences is unknown. Collagen alpha-chains are synthesized as a pro-alpha-chains, with globular extensions at both ends of the helical region. There is further evidence indicating that a pre-peptide, required for intracellular membrane passage, is clipped before secretion.

The hydroxylation of proline and lysine residues begins before completion of the chain and continues during passage of the newly formed chains through the rough endoplasmic reticulum. The respective hydroxylases require ascorbic acid as a cofactor. Glycosylation of hydroxylysine hydroxyl groups also occurs at this stage, as does asparagine (N-linked) glycosylation of the pro-peptides.

Triple helix formation is also believed to occur within the endoplasmic reticulum. The carboxy-terminal pro-peptides associate first, forming interchain disulfide bonds, after which the process extends rapidly along the molecule to the amino-terminal pro-peptide. The molecules then pass through intermediate vacuoles to the Golgi apparatus, where further processing may occur, after which they are secreted.

The conversion of pro-collagen to collagen, i.e., clipping of the amino-terminal and carboxy-terminal pro-peptides, occurs after secretion of the molecule into the extracellular space. Aggregation of collagen molecules into microfibrils then follows. This appears, under physiological conditions, to be a spontaneous process. The nonhelical ends of the alpha-chains appear to be essential for fibril formation. This molecular aggregation is subsequently rendered irreversible by cross-linking of the collagen molecules. The latter is preceded by oxidative deamination of lysine residues with the formation of aldehydes, which may then react in a variety of ways to form covalent inter-molecular cross links.

The regulation of collagen synthesis is imperfectly understood. It has been shown that collagen synthesis is a highly conserved property of cultured cells, persisting throughout the life of the cell and through repeated subcultures. Interstitial collagens are synthesized by fibroblasts, which usually produce collagen types I and III in a ratio of approximately 9:1. There has been some controversy as to the extent to which this synthesis ratio is maintained by different cell types. Thus, some investigators have shown the type I:type III synthesis ratio to be highly conserved, whereas others have shown variability with different culture conditions.

A variety of factors have been shown to influence collagen synthesis, both quantitatively and qualitatively, at the cellular level. These factors include viral transformation, phorbol esters, bromodeoxyuridine, ascorbic acid, iron chelators, etc. A factor that may be of particular importance as a physiological regulator is the amino-terminal pro-peptide. This has been shown to inhibit collagen synthesis and may thus function as a feedback regulator.

Collagen Degradation

Collagens are extremely resistant to degradation by proteolytic enzymes. Type 3 collagen is sensitive to trypsin and neutrophil elastase. In general, however, collagens are degraded only by collagenases. Bacterial collagenases are relatively nonspecific in their cleavage site, being active between triplets consisting of (Gly-X-Y) where X and Y may be proline or hydroxyproline.

Animal collagenase is widely distributed throughout the animal kingdom and cleaves between residues 772 and 773 (glycine and isoleucine) in the alpha 1(I) chain and at homologous sites in the alpha 1(II) and alpha 1(III) chains. This cleavage exposes the chain to the action of other proteases. Neutrophil elastase cleaves type III collagen at the same site, although the trypsin cleavage site is distinct. Neutrophils also produce a unique collagenase with far greater activity against type I collagen than type III.

The regulation of collagenase activity is complex and poorly understood. The enzyme is produced by a wide variety of cells, including endotoxin-stimulated macrophages, synovial cells, fibroblasts, and chondrocytes. Its synthesis is influenced by interactions both with other cells and the surrounding extracellular matrix. Mononuclear phagocytes have recently been shown to produce a factor that greatly enhances collagenase synthesis.

THE HISTOCHEMISTRY OF COLLAGEN

The word "collagen" literally refers to a substance that gives rise to glue. Early histochemists detected collagen in tissue by extraction into hot aqueous solution, which was followed by gelation on cooling. This resulted from denaturation of collagen to gelatin, which is more readily soluble. The use of trichrome stains, such as those of Mallory, Masson, Van Gieson, etc., for the detection of collagen did not become standard practice until the end of the 19th century.

Koelliker, in 1854, described a fibrous material in loose connective tissue that did not yield gelatin on extraction (6); he therefore proposed that the latter was biochemically distinct from collagen. It was later demonstrated in 1892, by Young (7), that early failures to obtain gelatin from loose connective tissues resulted from the use of excessive volumes of water in the extraction procedure and that the simple expedient of reducing the extraction volume increased the concentration of gelatin to the extent that gelation was possible. It was therefore concluded that fine connective tissue fibers were composed of collagen. This did not, however, resolve the controversy.

Bielschowsky, in 1904, described a silver impregnation technique for the demonstration of neurofibrils (8), and this was later shown by Maresch (9) to stain a variety of fine connective tissue fibers, as well as epithelial basement membranes. Although Maresch himself never suggested that silver impregnation was specific for any particular connective tissue component, this misconception appears to have slipped into the literature. Thus, fine connective tissue fibers, or "reticular" fibers, were believed to be composed of a protein, reticulin, that was distinct from collagen. This latter material was detectable by silver impregnation—a supposedly specific stain for a supposedly specific protein (10). This totally unfounded belief remains widespread to the present day.

There is no rational basis, therefore, for the distinction between collagen fibrosis and reticulin fibrosis. In both cases, the fibrous protein deposited in the extracellular space is collagen, which is now definable in precise, biochemical terms. The nature of the reactive material stained by silver impregnation remains a matter of debate. It is certain, however, that the latter is not collagen. This question has been reviewed at length by Puchtler and Waldrop (11), who suggest that it may be a soluble polysaccharide or glycoprotein, associated with fine connective tissue fibers and basement membranes.

Recent developments in collagen biochemistry have enabled the preparation of pure collagens, which have been used to raise specific antisera (12). Thus, it is now possible to localize and identify collagens in tissue sections by immunohistochemical techniques. This has led to new insights into collagen histochemistry within a variety of organs, including the bone marrow.

CONNECTIVE TISSUE ELEMENTS IN BONE MARROW

Bone marrow, like other tissues, has a well-defined connective tissue structure. The major cellular component of bone marrow connective tissue is the reticular cell. The latter is visible in electron micrographs as a large cell, with branching cytoplasm, that is intimately associated with the meshwork of fine connective tissue fibers that form the supporting structure of the bone marrow. Reticular cells are distributed throughout the hematopoietic compartment of the marrow and clothe the abluminal surfaces of the marrow sinusoids (13, 14).

There is strong evidence to indicate that reticular cells are fibroblastic. Cells of similar morphology and distribution thus are demonstrable by immunofluorescence, using specific anti-collagen antibodies, in frozen sections of bone marrow (15). These cells are ubiquitous throughout the hematopoietic space and are closely related to an extracellular collagenous meshwork that is so extensive as to surround virtually every individual cell. Material stained for type I and type III collagens show identical appearances, indicating that both types of collagen are synthesized by individual reticular cells.

Another important property of bone marrow reticular cells is their tendency, under certain circumstances, to accumulate intracellular lipid (13, 14), giving rise to the fat spaces normally observed within the marrow cavity. The mechanism by which this occurs is not understood and its significance remains obscure. The tendency to lipogenesis is also manifest in vitro by marrow-derived fibroblastoid cells and has been shown to be biochemically distinct from lipogenesis in adipose tissues elsewhere. In particular, the process is corticosteroid-sensitive and insulin-resistant (16).

Biochemical studies of bone marrow cells in short-term culture indicate the synthesis of small, but detectable quantities of collagen types I and III

(15, 17). The ratio of type I:type III collagen synthesis was approximately 5:1. It was of interest to note that this type I:type III ratio was conserved during cultivation of marrow connective tissue cells under conditions known to be associated with long-term maintenance of hematopoietic stem cells in vitro (18).

There is evidence to suggest that marrow connective tissue, or stromal elements provide functional, as well as structural support for hematopoiesis. Marrow hematopoietic elements are destroyed by irradiation to 700 rads, but stromal elements are spared and hematopoiesis may be reestablished by transplantation of suitable donor marrow cells. Supralethal irradiation, however, to a level of 1500 rads, destroys both marrow hematopoietic and stromal elements and transplanted marrow cells fail to engraft (19). Mechanical damage resulting from curettage of the marrow cavity is ultimately followed by reestablishment of hematopoiesis, but the latter is invariably preceded by the development of a stromal architecture (20). A similar sequence of events follows transplantation of marrow fragments to extramedullary sites (21).

Studies of this kind provide strong circumstantial evidence implicating marrow stromal elements as mediators of the hematopoietic microenvironment. More direct evidence has been derived from in vitro marrow culture techniques (see below).

STUDIES OF MARROW STROMAL CELLS IN VITRO

To study the biology of bone marrow stroma, a number of authors have attempted to cultivate stromal cells from primary explants of bone marrow. In fact, early attempts at bone marrow culture (22) resulted almost invariably in the growth of marrow stromal rather than hematopoietic elements.

The first serious attempt to characterize marrow connective tissue cells in vitro was made by Friedenstein et al. (23). Guinea pig marrow cells were explanted in TC-199 with 20% fetal calf serum. Colonies of stromal cells were apparent 3 days after explantation, reaching confluence at 2–3 weeks. These cells had the appearance of fibroblasts and were stainable by trichrome collagen stains and by silver impregnation. The colonies were shown to be clonal in nature (24).

On transplantation beneath the renal capsules of syngeneic recipients, these cells induced the formation of ossicles that subsequently became populated by hematopoietic bone marrow (25). The hematopoietic elements in this ectopic hematopoietic tissue were found to be of recipient origin, but the stromal elements were shown to be derived from the transplanted fibroblastic cells (26). These results suggest a remarkable potential for marrow stromal cells as regulators of bone marrow growth.

Other attempts at cultivation of marrow stromal cells in liquid culture systems resulted in the growth of more heterogeneous layers of marrow-derived adherent cells (MDAC). Thus, Zipori and Bol (27) observed two cell types in their MDAC cultures, with morphological characteristics suggesting the presence of fibroblasts and macrophages. The "macrophages" exhibited phagocytic activity against latex particles, whereas this property was less pronounced in the "fibroblasts." Density separation suggested that these two cell types arose from different precursors. Essentially similar heterogeneity was observed by Werts et al. (28). The majority of MDAC in the latter system were large, polygonal cells, staining positively with Masson's trichrome stain. The remaining cells were actively phagocytic and stained positively for nonspecific esterase.

Collagen synthesis by bone marrow stromal elements in vitro was first confirmed using objective techniques by Castro-Malaspina et al. (29). MDAC were cultivated in TC-199 medium with 20% fetal calf serum and the resulting colonies of adherent cells appeared similar to those described by Friedenstein et al. (23). Immunofluorescent staining for collagen types I and III indicated that collagens of both types were synthesized. These cultures appeared to be homogeneously composed of fibroblasts, without evidence of any other cell type.

Perhaps the most significant observed property of MDAC is their capacity, under appropriate culture conditions, to support the proliferation of hematopoietic stem cells for prolonged periods in vitro. The long-term bone marrow culture (LTBMC) system, first described by Dexter et al. (18), involved primary culture of MDAC layers from mouse marrow cells explanted in Fischer's medium with 25% horse serum. The culture system was critically dependent upon the use of suitable batches of horse serum. Confluent MDAC cultures were then recharged with second explants of marrow cells and subsequently fed by removing half the culture supernatant and replacing it with fresh medium. Under these conditions, it was possible to maintain stem cell proliferation for many months.

The dependence of this system on horse serum was later shown to be the result of a requirement for hydrocortisone, to the extent that the latter was shown to restore the capacity of defective batches of horse serum to support in vitro hematopoiesis (16). The MDAC layer in LTBMC was found to be morphologically heterogeneous, including fibroblastoid cells, phagocytic mononuclear cells, epithelioid cells, and adipocytes (18). Cultures that were successful in terms of long-term hematopoietic support were found to contain large numbers of adipocytes, and lipogenesis within the adherent layer was induced by hydrocortisone supplementation. In cultures supporting active hematopoiesis, these layers also included a variety of hematopoietic elements.

In studies of actively hematopoietic cultures, the adherent layers were so heterogeneous that it was difficult to distinguish stromal from hematopoietic elements (4, 30-31). Far less was it possible to identify the particular stromal elements responsible for long-term stem cell maintenance. Studies of unrecharged, potentially hematopoietic MDAC layers, however, indicate that fibroblastic cells, synthesizing collagen types I and III, were by far the major population (17, 32-33).

This does not necessarily mean that marrow fibroblasts, per se, provide the permissive microenvironment required for the maintenance of hematopoiesis in vivo or in vitro. Marrow fibroblasts, cultured under a variety of conditions (22-29) are incapable of supporting in vitro hematopoiesis. Similarly, fibroblastoid cell lines derived from LTBMC (34, 35) are microenvironmentally incompetent.

THE ORIGIN OF MARROW STROMA

This has been the subject of considerable debate. MDAC have been shown to resemble reticular cells in a number of respects. Thus reticular cells, like MDAC, stain by immunofluorescence for interstitial collagens (types I and III), and are closely associated with an extensive extracellular matrix of collagen fibers distributed throughout the hematopoietic compartment of the bone marrow (16). The capacity of reticular cells in intact bone marrow to accumulate lipid under certain conditions has already been mentioned (15). These similarities provide good circumstantial evidence suggesting that MDAC in vitro are derived either from mature reticular cells or from their precursors. The hematopoietic microenvironments in vivo and in vitro would thus appear to be mediated by similar cellular elements.

The developmental relationship between hematopoietic cells and microenvironmental elements is less well established. Many studies have been performed on bone marrow fibroblasts (36-44), but these cells cannot be regarded as microenvironmentally competent. Although certain authors present evidence suggesting that marrow fibroblasts are derived from hematopoietic stem cells (36, 37), the majority of studies (38-44) support the opposite conclusion.

Only two studies have addressed directly the question of the origin of the stromal elements in LTBMC. Bentley et al. (45) reconstituted lethally irradiated mice with murine marrow cells bearing the T6 chromosome marker. MDAC were then cultivated using marrow explants from these transplanted mice. The proportion of T6 positive mitoses progressively declined during the cultivation period and at the time of confluence (6 weeks after explantation), the only mitoses detectable were T6 negative (recipient). This would suggest that MDAC precursors were not transplantable and were not, therefore, derived from HSC.

Keating et al. (4) prepared LTBMCs from human subjects who had received marrow transplants from donors of the opposite sex. Using fluorescent Y-body analysis, these authors were able to demonstrate that marrow stromal elements were of donor origin and therefore transplantable. Although no simple explanation can be offered for these apparently contradictory findings, a number of possibilities have been discussed.

In the study of Bentley et al. (45), recipient animals were prepared for transplantation by radiation only and relatively small numbers of cells were infused (10^5 cells per mouse). In the study of Keating et al. (4), patients were pretreated with a combination of total body irradiation and cyclophosphamide. It is possible that the latter drug "punched holes" in the stromal structure of the marrow and enabled donor stromal elements, which were infused in very large numbers, to colonize the marrow space (46).

There remains the question of whether donor-type stromal elements were derived from transplanted stromal elements or from transplanted stem cells. Singer et al. (47) have presented evidence from patients with clonal myeloproliferative disorders suggesting that stromal elements in LTBMC may indeed be derived from stem cells. This concept of a developmental relationship between blood and connective tissue is by no means a novel one, having been proposed by Maximow (48) 55 years ago. The evidence, however, is conflicting. The possibility remains that bone marrow connective tissue cells may, under appropriate conditions, be derived both from stem cells and from nonhematopoietic marrow cells.

FIBROSIS IN THE MYELOPROLIFERATIVE SYNDROMES

Study of the myeloproliferative disorders was greatly enhanced by the development of techniques for investigating the clonality of cell populations. The first clonal markers to be studied were cytogenetic and a major advance was the demonstration that a specific chromosomal abnormality, the Ph1 chromosome (49, 50), was demonstrable.

Of particular importance in the study of myelofibrosis was the development of a technique for the investigation of clonality that did not depend on cellular proliferation or the presence of a chromosome marker. Such a technique is based upon glucose-6-phosphate dehydrogenase (G6PD) isoenzyme analysis (51). The applicability of this technique is limited to females who are heterozygous for a G6PD variant, but a number of such patients have been studied. These studies indicate that marrow fibroblasts in myelofibrosis are developmentally distinct from the hematopoietic population (3). Fibrosis must therefore be regarded as a reaction to a primary stem cell proliferation.

This view is supported by the observation that cultivated, marrow-derived fibroblasts in myelofibrosis are phenotypically normal with respect to a variety of characteristics, including their proliferative capacity and rate of collagen synthesis (52). Further evidence for the latter conclusion is provided by the findings in a case of myelofibrosis treated by bone marrow transplantation (55). Successful engraftment of normal hematopoietic elements was associated with regression of marrow fibrosis.

The mechanisms whereby stem cell proliferation leads to increased deposition of collagen fiber remain hypothetical, although the subject has been reviewed at length by Castro-Malaspina et al. (53, 54). The amount of collagen within a tissue would be determined by the number of collagen-producing cells, the rate of collagen synthesis by individual cells, and the rate of collagen catabolism.

The number of collagen-producing cells within the marrow would depend primarily upon their proliferative state in vivo. Much attention has therefore been focused upon the possibility that hematopoietic cells might produce factors that stimulate bone marrow fibroblast growth. The prime candidate for this role is platelet-derived growth factor (PGDF), a substance present in platelet alpha-granules that stimulates the growth of a variety of cell types, including fibroblasts (56). A similar growth factor has been identified in megakaryocytes (57).

Megakaryocytic proliferation is a prominent feature of myelofibrosis, and the marrow frequently contains large numbers of morphologically abnormal megakaryocytes (58). Quantitative histomorphometric studies of marrow fiber production in this disorder (59) have demonstrated that a correlation exists between the peripheral platelet count and the extent of marrow fibrosis in splenectomized patients with myelofibrosis. This would suggest a relationship between megakaryopoietic and fibroblastic activity. Ineffective megakaryopoiesis, with intramedullary death of megakaryocytes and release of growth factors, has been proposed as a possible underlying cause of fibroblastic proliferation in myelofibrosis (53, 54) and remains the most plausible model currently available.

However, the role of PDGF as mediator of the fibrotic reaction that occurs in myelofibrosis is by no means established. It must be remembered that the disorder is characterized by replacement of the entire hematopoietic tissue by a neoplastic clone and that candidate growth factors may be produced by other cell types. Factors derived from monocyte-macrophages and from T lymphocytes may also be significant in this respect (60).

Another potentially important mechanism for increased bone marrow collagen in myelofibrosis is failure of the normal catabolic process. Castro-Malaspina et al. (53, 54) incorporate this possibility into their ineffective megakaryopoiesis model. Citing observations that platelet factor 4 inhibits collagenase activity (61), they suggest that such inhibition may contribute to the pathogenesis of myelofibrosis, but is unlikely to be the primary lesion. Further possibilities relate to defective collagenase synthesis by neutrophils in myelofibrosis and failure of monocytes to secrete factors that stimulate collagenase synthesis. None of these possibilities has been investigated.

COMMENTARY

It will be evident from this review of recent literature that an abundance of data has been obtained that may be of significance in elucidating the pathogenesis of myelofibrosis. Unfortunately, much of the available evidence is conflicting, and cautious interpretation is essential. It goes without saying, in the current stage of knowledge, that no firm conclusions can be drawn.

The greatest single source of confusion in this area is the bone marrow fibroblast. The fibroblast phenotype is poorly defined and no distinctive marker has been identified. The synthesis of collagens type I and type III is a general property of fibroblasts, but this property is shared by a variety of other cell phenotypes. Moreover, the differences between fibroblastic connective tissue cells cultivated from different organs or tissues are poorly documented, as is the extent to which the in vivo characteristics of fibroblasts are maintained in vitro, especially after repeated subculture. Any conclusions derived from studies of bone marrow fibroblasts, therefore, must be regarded as tentative.

An essential question is whether the various phenotypes observed among marrow-derived connective tissue cells in different tissue culture systems reflect selection of different phenotypes from the parent population or variability within a single population resulting from differences in culture conditions. The major connective tissue element within the hematopoietic tissue is the reticular cell, as described above, but hematopoietic tissue is not homogeneous and contains vascular and neural elements in addition to blood-forming cells. These structures include connective tissue elements that are distinct from those of the hematopoietic tissue. Marrow is invariably enclosed within bone. The latter is surrounded by periosteum and lined by endosteum, both of which are composed of fibrous connective tissue. The origin of a particular culture of marrow-derived fibroblasts cannot, therefore, in the present state of knowledge, be identified with certainty.

It has been convincingly established that hematopoietic elements in myelofibrosis (3), as in other myeloproliferative disorders (51), are clonally derived and must, therefore, be regarded as neoplastic. As previously discussed, the weight of evidence, at least numerically, would lead to the conclusion that marrow fibroblastic elements are derived from nonhematopoietic progenitor cells (38–44) rather than hematopoietic stem cells (36, 37). This, in turn, would support the conclusion that marrow fibrosis is a reaction to some factor, as yet undefined, that is produced by the hematopoietic clone.

Investigations into the origin of marrow stroma, however, have invariably involved the cultivation of bone marrow fibroblasts, with the implicit assumption that the latter are truly representative of hematopoietic-associated connective tissue elements. This is by no means certain. Connective tissue elements in LTBMC are more likely to be derived from hematopoietic stroma, but the nonhomogeneity of MDAC in the latter system makes interpretation difficult. The present author (45) has presented data suggesting that connective tissue cells in LTBMC are developmentally distinct from hematopoietic stem cells, whereas Keating et al. (4, 46) present evidence suggesting the opposite conclusion.

The majority of investigators would favor the hypothesis that myelofibrosis represents the stromal reaction to a primary, clonal myeloproliferative disease. An alternative hypothesis could be advanced, based upon the concept of a common origin of bone marrow stromal and hematopoietic elements from hematopoietic stem cells. In such a hypothesis, it would be postulated that the syndrome results from stem cell proliferation with an exaggerated tendency for differentiation toward connective tissue cells. Although the weight of evidence militates strongly against such a conclusion, the latter cannot be totally excluded.

REFERENCES

1. Hueck, G. (1879). Zwei Falle von Leukamie mit eigenthumlichen Blut- resp. Knochenmarksbefund. *Virchows Arch.* (*Pathol. Anat.*) *78*: 475–479.
2. Damashek, W. (1951). Some speculations on the myeloproliferative disorders. *Blood 6*: 372–375.
3. Jacobson, R. J., Salo, A. and Fialkow, P. J. (1978). Agnogenic myeloid

metaplasia: A clonal proliferation of hematopoietic stem cells with secondary myelofibrosis. *Blood 51*: 189–194.

4. Keating, A., Singer, J. W., Killen, P. D., Striker, G. E., Salo, A. C., Sanders, J., Thomas, E. D., Thorning, D., and Fialkow, P. J. (1982). Donor origin of the hematopoietic microenvironment after marrow transplantation in man. *Nature 298*: 280–283.
5. Bornstein, P., and Traub, W. (1979). The chemistry and biology of collagen. In *The Proteins*, H. Neurath and R. L. Hill (Eds.), volume IV, New York, Academic Press, pp. 412–524.
6. Koelliker, A. (1854). *Manual of Human Microscopic Anatomy*, J. da Costa (Ed.), Philadelphia, Lippincott, Grambo and Co.
7. Young, R. A. (1892). The fibres of retiform tissue. *J. Physiol. 13*: 332–334.
8. Bielschowsky, M. (1904). Die silberimpregnation der Neurofibrillen. *J. Psych. Neurol. 3*: 169–189.
9. Maresch, R. (1905). Uber Gitterfasern der Leber und die Verwendbarkeit der Methode Bielschowskys zur Darstellung feinster Bindegewebsfibrillen. *Zentralbl. Alg. Path. path. Anat. 16*: 641–649.
10. Foot, N. C. (1928). Chemical contrasts between collagenous and reticular connective tissue. *Am. J. Pathol. 4*: 525–544.
11. Puchtler, H. and Waldrop, F. S. (1978). Silver impregnation methods for reticulum fibers and reticulin: a reinvestigation of their origins and specificity. *Histochemistry 57*: 177–187.
12. Gay, S., Fietzek, P. P., Remberger, K., Eder, M., and Kuhn, K. (1975). Liver cirrhosis: immunofluorescence and biochemical studies demonstrate two types of collagen. *Klin. Woch. 53*: 205–208.
13. Weiss, L. (1975). The hematopoietic microenvironment of the bone marrow. An ultrastructural study of the stroma in rats. *Anat. Rec. 186*: 161–184.
14. Lichtman, M. D. (1981). The ultrastructure of the hemopoietic environment of the marrow: a review. *Exp. Hematol. 9*: 391–410.
15. Bentley, S. A., Foidart, J.-M., and Kleinman, H. K. (1984). Connective tissue elements in rat bone marrow: Immunofluorescent visualization of the hematopoietic microenvironment. *J. Histochem. Cytochem. 32*: 114–116.
16. Greenberger, J. S. (1978). Sensitivity of corticosteroid-dependent, insulin-resistant lipogenesis in marrow preadipocytes of mutation diabetic-obese mice. *Nature 275*: 752–753.
17. Bentley, S. A. (1982). Collagen synthesis by bone marrow stromal cells: a quantitative study. *Br. J. Haematol. 50*: 491–497.
18. Dexter, T. M., Allen, T. D., and Lajtha, L. G. (1977). Conditions controlling the proliferation of haemopoietic stem cells in vitro. *J. Cell. Physiol. 91*: 335–344.

19. Knospe, W. H., Blom, J., and Crosby, W. H. (1966). Regeneration of locally-irradiated bone marrow. I. Dose-dependent long-term changes in the rat with particular emphasis upon vascular and stromal reaction. *Blood 28*: 398–415.
20. Patt, H. M. and Moloney, M. A. (1970). Reconstitution of bone marrow in a depleted medullary cavity. In *Hemopoietic Cellular Proliferation*, F. Stohlman (Ed.), New York, Grune & Stratton, pp. 56–66.
21. Tavassoli, M. and Crosby, W. H. (1968). Transplantation of marrow to extramedullary sites. *Science 161*: 54–56.
22. Carrel, A. and Burrows, M. T. (1910). Culture de moelle osseux et de rate. *Comptes Rend. Soc. Biol. 69*: 299–311.
23. Friedenstein, A. J., Chailakhjan, R. K., and Lalykin, K. S. (1970). The development of fibroblast colonies in monolayer cultures of guinea pig bone marrow and spleen cells. *Cell. Tissue Kinet. 3*: 393–403.
24. Friedenstein, A. J., Deriglasova, U. F., Kulagina, N. N., Panasuk, A. F., Rudakowa, E. E., Luria, E. A., and Rudakow, I. A. (1974). Precursors for fibroblasts in different populations of hematopoietic cells as determined by the in vitro colony assay method. *Exp. Hematol. 2*: 83–92.
25. Friedenstein, A. J., Chailakhyan, R. K., Latsinik, N. V., Panaysuk, A. F., and Keiliss-Borok, I. V. (1974). Stromal cells responsible for transferring the microenvironment of the hemopoietic tissues. *Transplantation 17*: 331–340.
26. Friedenstein, A. J., Ivanov-Smolenski, A. A., Chailakhjan, R. K., Gorskaya, V. F., Kuralesova, A. I., Latzinik, N. W., and Gerasimow, V. W. (1978). Origin of bone marrow stromal mechanocytes in radiochimeras and heterotopic transplants. *Exp. Hematol. 6*: 440–444.
27. Zipori, D. and Bol, S. (1979). The role of fibroblastoid cells and macrophages from mouse bone marrow in the in vivo growth promotion of haemopoietic tumour cells. *Exp. Hematol. 7*: 206–218.
28. Werts, E. D., de Gowin, R. L., Knapp, S. K., and Gibson, D. P. (1980). Characterization of marrow stromal (fibroblastoid) cells and their association with erythropoiesis. *Exp. Hematol. 8*: 423–433.
29. Castro-Malaspina, H., Gay, R. E., Resnick, G., Kapoor, N., Meyers, P., Chiarieri, D., McKenzie, S., Broxmeyer, H. E., and Moore, M. A. A. (1980). Characterization of human bone marrow fibroblast colony-forming units (CFU-F) and their progeny. *Blood 56*: 289–301.
30. Castro-Malaspina, H., Gay, R. E., Saletan, S., Oettgen, B., Gay, S., and Moore, M. A. S. (1981). Phenotypic characterization of the adherent cell layer in long-term mouse bone marrow cultures. *Blood 5(Suppl. 1)*: 107a.
31. Zuckerman, K. S. and Wicha, M. S. (1983). Extracellular matrix production by the adherent cells of long-term murine bone marrow cultures. *Blood 61*: 540–547.
32. Bentley, S. A. and Foidart, J-M. (1980). Some properties of marrow derived adherent cells in tissue culture. *Blood 56*: 1006–1012.

33. Bentley, S. A. and Tralka, T. S. (1982). Characterization of marrow-derived adherent cells: evidence against an endothelial subpopulation. *Scand. J. Haematol. 28*: 381–388.
34. Harigaya, K., Cronkite, E. D., Miller, M. E., and Shadduck, R. E. (1981). Murine bone marrow cell line producing colony-stimulating factor. *Proc. Natl. Acad. Sci., U.S.A. 78*: 6963–6966.
35. Lanotte, M., Sectt, D., Dexter, T. M., and Allen, T. D. (1982). Clonal preadipocyte cell lines with different phenotypes derived from murine marrow stroma: factors influencing growth and adipogenesis in vitro. *J. Cell. Physiol. 111*: 177–186.
36. Hentel, J. and Hirschhorn, K. (1971). The origin of some bone marrow fibroblasts. *Blood 38*: 81–86.
37. Lozzio, C. B., Lozzio, B. B., Wust, C. J., and Kim, J. (1978). Correlation of leukemia associated antigens and Phl chromosome in fibroblast like cells derived from human bone marrow. *Blood 52*: 673–680.
38. Maniatis, A. K., Amsel, S., Mitus, W. J., and Coleman, N. (1969). Chromosome pattern of bone marrow fibroblasts in patients with chronic granulocytic leukemia. *Nature 222*: 1278–1279.
39. van Slyck, E. J., Weiss, L., and Dully, M. (1970). Chromosomal evidence for the secondary role of bone marrow fibroblast proliferation in acute myelofibrosis. *Blood 36*: 729–735.
40. Friedenstein, A. J. and Kuralesova, A. I. (1971). Osteogeneic precursor cells of bone marrow in radiation chimeras. *Transplantation 12*: 99–108.
41. de la Chapelle, A., Vuopio, P., and Borgstrom, H. (1973). The origin of bone marrow fibroblasts. *Blood 41*: 783–787.
42. Wilson, F. D., Greenberg, B. R., Konrad, P. N., Klein, A. K., and Walling, P. A. (1978). Cytogenetic studies on bone marrow fibroblasts from a male-female hematopoietic chimera. Evidence that stromal elements in human transplantation are of host type. *Transplantation 25*: 87–88.
43. Greenberg, B. R., Wilson, F. D., Woo, L., and Jenks, H. M. (1978). Cytogenetics of fibroblast colonies in Phl positive chronic myelogenous leukemia. *Blood 51*: 1039–1044.
44. Golde, D. W., Hocking, W. G., Quan, S. G., Sparkes, R. S., and Gale, R. P. (1980). Origin of human bone marrow fibroblasts. *Br. J. Haematol. 44*: 183–187.
45. Bentley, S. A., Knutsen, T., and Whang-Peng, J. (1982). The origin of the hematopoietic microenvironment in continuous bone marrow culture. *Exp. Hematol. 10*: 367–372.
46. Singer, J. W., Keating, A., and Fialkow, P. J. (1983). Evidence suggesting a common progenitor for hematopoietic and marrow stromal cells. *Exp. Hematol. 11(Suppl. 14)*: 4.
47. Dexter, T. M. (1982). Is the marrow stroma transplantable? *Nature 298*: 222–223.
48. Maximow, A. A. (1928). Cultures of blood leucocytes. From lympho-

cyte and monocyte to connective tissue. *Arch. Exp. Zellforsch. 5*: 169–182.

49. Nowell, P. C. and Hungerford, D. A. (1960). A minute chromosome in human chronic granulocytic leukemia. *Science 132*: 1497–1499.
50. Whang, J., Frei, E., Tjio, J. H., Carbone, P. P., and Brecher, G. (1963). The distribution of the Philadelphia chromosome in patients with chronic myelocytic leukemia. *Blood 22*: 664–673.
51. Adamson, J. W. and Fialkow, P. J. (1978). The pathogenesis of the myeloproliferative syndromes. *Br. J. Haematol. 38*: 299–303.
52. Castro-Malaspina, H., Gay, R. E., Jhanwar, S. C., Hamilton, J. A., Chiarieri, D., Meyers, P. A., Gay, S., and Moore, M. A. S. (1982). Characteristics of bone marrow fibroblast colony-forming cells (CFU-F) and their progeny in myeloproliferative disorders. *Blood 59*: 1046–1054.
53. Castro-Malaspina, H. and Moore, M. A. S. (1982). Pathophysiological mechanisms operating in the development of myelofibrosis: role of megakaryocytes. *Nouv. Rev. Fr. Hematol. 24*: 221–224.
54. Castro-Malaspina, H. (1984). Pathogenesis of myelofibrosis: role of ineffective megakaryopoiesis and megakaryocyte components. In *Myelofibrosis and the Biology of Connective Tissue*, P. D. Berk, H. Castro-Malaspina and L. R. Wasserman (Eds.), Alan R. Liss, Inc., New York, pp. 427–454.
55. Rappeport, J., Parkman, R., Belli, J., Levey, R., Rosen, F., and Nathan, D. (1978). Reversibility of myelofibrosis after bone marrow transplantation. *Blood 52* (*Suppl. 1*): 598.
56. Kaplan, D. R., Chao, F. C., Stiles, C. D., Antoniades, H. N., and Scher, C. D. (1979). Platelet alpha-granules contain a growth factor for fibroblasts. *Blood 53*: 1043–1052.
57. Castro-Malaspina, H., Rabellino, E. M., Yen, A., Nachman, R. L., and Moore, M. A. S. (1981). Human megakaryocyte stimulation of proliferation of bone marrow fibroblasts. *Blood 57*: 781–786.
58. Ward, H. P. and Block, M. H. (1971). The natural history of agnogenic myeloid metaplasia (AMM) and a critical evaluation of its relationship to the myeloproliferative syndrome. *Medicine 50*: 357–420.
59. Bentley, S. A. and Herman, C. J. (1979). Bone marrow fibre production in myelofibrosis: a quantitative study. *Br. J. Haematol. 42*: 51–59.
60. Wahl, S. M. (1984). Lymphocyte and macrophage derived fibroblast growth factors. In *Myelofibrosis and the Biology of Connective Tissue*, P. D. Berk, H. Castro-Malaspina and L. R. Wasserman (Eds.), Alan R. Liss, Inc., New York, p. 143–154.
61. Hiti-Harper, J., Wohl, H., and Harper, E. (1978). Platelet factor 4: an inhibitor of collagenase. *Science 199*: 991–993.

5

Hematopoietic Progenitor Cells in Myelofibrosis

JILL A. HIBBIN AND JOHN M. GOLDMAN
Royal Postgraduate Medical School, Hammersmith Hospital, London, England

INTRODUCTION

Primary myelofibrosis (PMF) has been classified as a myeloproliferative disorder (1, 2) along with polycythemia rubra vera (PV), essential thrombocythemia (ET), and chronic granulocytic leukemia (CGL). Marrow fibrosis is an essential feature of PMF but it may also occur in the other myeloproliferative disorders and in other conditions, including Hodgkin's disease, carcinoma metastatic to bone marrow, and tuberculosis.

There is evidence that the marrow fibrosis in PMF is a reaction to disturbed hemopoiesis. Van Slyck et al. (3) showed that the blood cells from a patient with acute myelofibrosis had a consistent chromosomal abnormality, whereas the bone marrow fibroblasts had normal karyotypes. Khan et al. (4) and Jacobson et al. (5) showed that in patients heterozygous for the A and B isoenzymes of glucose-6-phosphate dehydrogenase (G6PD), the bone marrow fibroblasts expressed both isoenzymes but the blood cells only expressed one type. These observations suggested that the blood cells in this disorder are clonally derived and therefore presumably malignant, whereas the marrow fibroblasts are normal. Further evidence for the "reactive" nature of the fibrosis comes from the successful reversal of the fibrosis following allogeneic bone marrow transplantation (6–8).

HEMATOPOIETIC PROGENITOR CELL ASSAYS

Granulocyte/Macrophage Progenitor Cells

In 1971 Pike and Robinson (9) modified the murine method developed by Bradley and Metcalf (10) to permit growth in agar of colonies of cells from human bone marrow. Underlayers of leukocytes were used as feeder layers to provide humoral factors needed for the growth of the colonies. The numbers of colonies produced were proportional to the number of bone marrow cells plated, indicating that the colonies were derived from single cells. The progenitor cells giving rise to these colonies were initially known as CFU-C (colony-forming unit in culture). The colonies consisted of granulocytes and/or macrophages and are now known as CFU-GM to indicate their commitment to granulocyte/macrophage differentiation. Feeder layers have since been replaced by medium conditioned by various different human tissues, the most commonly used being mitogen- (usually phytohemagglutinin) stimulated lymphocytes. These conditioned media (CM) contain molecules known as colony-stimulating activity (CSA) or colony-stimulating factors (CSF). Some of these factors have been purified and shown to stimulate the growth of different colony types (11).

Erythroid Progenitor Cells

Tepperman et al. (12) adapted a plasma clot system, previously described by Stephenson et al. (13) and McLeod et al. (14), to grow colonies of hemoglobin-synthesizing cells from human bone marrow. They suggested that there were at least two populations of erythroid progenitors, a more mature CFU-E (colony-forming unit, erythroid) and a less mature cell analogous with the BFU-E (burst-forming unit, erythroid) found in mouse bone marrow. Iscove et al. (15) developed a methyl cellulose assay system for growing BFU-E and suggested that the erythroid CSA that they used was in fact erythropoietin (Epo), a hormone known to stimulate red cell production in vivo (16). Clark and Housman (17) showed that the BFU-E were also present in normal peripheral blood.

Megakaryocyte Progenitor Cells

Vainchenker et al. (18, 19) used a plasma clot system and obtained growth of megakaryocyte (Mk) colonies from normal human bone marrow and peripheral blood. They found various sources of Epo to be good stimulators but also suggested that other factors must be necessary for optimal colony numbers. Maturation of the Mk and platelet shedding were normal, but the assay required plating of large numbers of cells.

Messner et al. (20) described a methyl cellulose system for growing Mk colonies using human plasma instead of fetal calf serum. They showed that human serum was inhibitory, as did Vainchenker et al. (21), and also found Epo was not necessary. Williams and Levine (22) proposed that megakaryocytopoiesis was controlled by two factors in vitro, Mk-CSA and thrombopoietin, both of which were necessary for optimal colony formation: Mk-CSA stimulated population expansion by stimulating CFU-Mk division, whereas thrombopoietin amplified platelet production by stimulating development of individual Mk.

Multilineage Progenitor Cells

Fauser and Messner (23) identified individual colonies consisting of Mk, macrophages, and eosinophils as well as neutrophils and erythroblasts. They used a methyl cellulose system with the addition of Epo and phytohemagglutinin-stimulated, lymphocyte-conditioned medium (PHA-LCM). The method was improved by Ash et al. (24) who showed that these mixed colony-forming cells were present in higher concentration in the bone marrow than in the blood of normal individuals, that they required less Epo than BFU-E, and that they had some self-replicating capacity. These progenitors are known as CFU-GEMM or CFU-mix and fulfill some of the criteria for a pluripotential stem cell. The assay system allows growth of the earliest progenitor cell that can be detected to date by in vitro methods.

GRANULOCYTE/MACROPHAGE PROGENITORS IN MYELOFIBROSIS (MF)

Chervenick (25) showed that patients with PMF had increased numbers of CFU-GM circulating in their peripheral blood; this finding has since been confirmed by others (26-32) (Fig. 1). Goldman et al. (27) found a correlation between circulating CFU-GM numbers and the peripheral blood leukocyte count, but Hibbin et al. (32) were unable to confirm the correlation in their patients. It has been shown that patients with MF secondary to other diseases (SMF) also had increased circulating CFU-GM numbers. Wang et al. (34) studied patients with PMF or SMF and compared them with normal individuals. They showed highest numbers of circulating CFU-GM in those patients with PMF; CFU-GM numbers in the SMF patients were somewhat lower, but

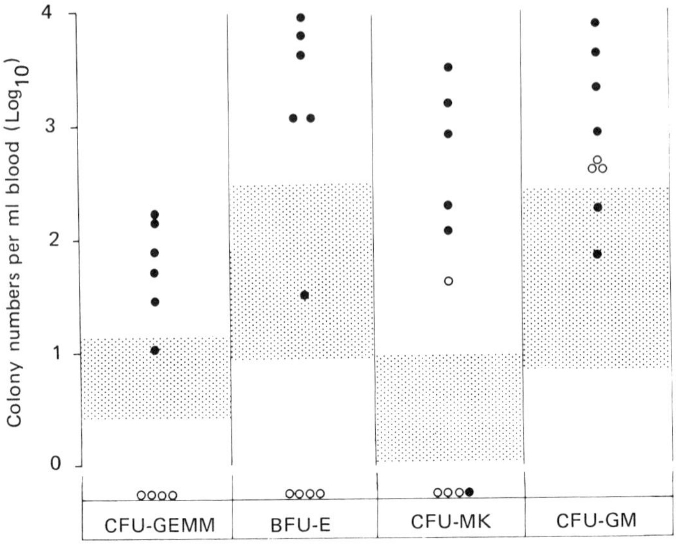

Figure 1 Progenitor cell numbers in the blood of patients with PMF and normal controls. Colony numbers are expressed on a log scale. In some patients, CFU-Mk numbers were increased by a factor of > 100. (●) Not splenectomized; (○) postsplenectomy. Stippled areas represent ranges for normal peripheral blood. [Reproduced from Hibbin et al. (Ref. 32) with permission of the publishers.]

still higher than in normal individuals; the three groups all overlapped to some extent.

Croizat et al. (30) found that the majority of their patients with PMF had CFU-GM that could produce colonies in the absence of any added PHA-LCM. They suggested that there was a population of CFU-GM independent of or highly sensitive to regulatory factors in the PHA-LCM and that this population was greater in patients with PMF than in normal individuals.

Partanen et al. (29) suggested two possible explanations for the increased numbers of circulating progenitors: either the stem cell and progenitor cell compartments were enlarged due to lack of control of the abnormal clone or the progenitors might be released prematurely from the bone marrow or extramedullary sites. Wang et al. (34) also proposed that disruption of the marrow microvascular system could lead to inappropriate release of large number of stem cells into the circulation.

There have been very few studies on CFU-GM numbers in the bone marrow of patients with PMF because of the difficulty in obtaining marrow aspirates. Two groups, however, reported increased granulocyte progenitor numbers in the bone marrow cultured in diffusion chambers implanted into the peritoneal cavity of mice (26, 28).

ERYTHROID PROGENITORS IN MYELOFIBROSIS

Ohl et al. (26) and Chikkappa et al. (28) used diffusion chamber techniques to demonstrate increases in erythroid progenitor cell numbers in the blood and bone marrow of patients with MF compared with normal individuals. Partanen et al. (29) reported that 12 of 18 patients with PMF had circulating CFU-E, whereas no circulating CFU-E were found in normal individuals. This has also been observed in other myeloproliferative disorders (35). Increased circulating BFU-E numbers in patients with MF were reported by several groups (29, 31, 32) (Fig. 1). The increases ranged from 8- to 13-fold. Croizat et al. (30) and Hibbin et al. (32) found some patients without circulating BFU-E and the former authors found that the rest of the patients had normal numbers. The differing results probably reflect the heterogeneity of the disease and differences in culture methods. Partanen et al. (29) suggested that clinical status of the patient might also be important, though Hibbin et al. (32) found no correlation between BFU-E numbers and leukocyte or platelet counts, hemoglobin level, or clinical status. Partanen et al. (29) also showed no correlation between CFU-GM and BFU-E numbers in the same patient, a finding confirmed by Hibbin (unpublished observation), but they did find a positive linear correlation between CFU-E and BFU-E numbers.

The studies suggest in general that there is an increase in circulating erythroid progenitor cell numbers in patients with PMF but that it is less marked than the increase in CFU-GM; this has also been noted for patients with CGL (36). It is interesting that some authors have reported that a proportion of BFU-E and/or CFU-E from some patients with PMF proliferate to form colonies in the absence of any exogenous Epo, forming so-called endogenous or spontaneous colonies (29, 32, 37, 38). Others, however, found no PMF patients with endogenous BFU-E in their circulation (30, 39).

Endogenous erythroid colonies have frequently been demonstrated in the blood and bone marrow of patients with PV (35, 37–42). Zanjani et al. (41) added anti-Epo antibodies directly to their plasma clot culture and also exposed components of the clot system to anti-Epo antibodies prior to use; in both cases, endogenous colony numbers were greatly reduced. They concluded that these colonies were not independent of Epo, but rather hypersensitive to the small quantities of Epo present in the serum and citrated plasma used in their system, quantities that were too low to be detected in their bioassay. They added very small amounts of highly purified Epo and obtained more erythroid colonies; when they added a larger amount of Epo they obtained maximum colony numbers, which suggested that there were two populations of progenitors, one hypersensitive and the other with normal sensitivity to Epo. The normal population was larger than the hypersensitive one and the two populations could be clearly distinguished in their dose-response characteristics.

Casadevall et al. (42) confirmed that some of the erythroid progenitors in PV were hypersensitive to Epo using a methyl cellulose system in the presence and absence of serum. They found no endogenous colonies in the absence of serum, whereas they were present when serum was used. The hypersensitive progenitors were not a homogeneous population but varied in their sensitivity to Epo.

Kornberg et al. (39) demonstrated endogenous erythroid colony formation only in patients with PV or in the patients with myelofibrosis with previous PV. They suggested that the assay could be used to differentiate cases of PMF from cases of "spent" PV with fibrosis when there was no clear history of preceding PV. Others, however, have shown that at least some PMF patients have a population of erythroid progenitors that are hypersensitive to Epo (29, 32, 38). Endogenous erythroid colonies have also been reported in at least one case of ET (40). The different results obtained from various groups may reflect differing assay conditions or the heterogeneity in the disease, but it is interesting that Epo hypersensitive erythroid progenitors have been found in some cases of all the myeloproliferative disorders, suggesting that these disorders are closely related.

MEGAKARYOCYTE PROGENITORS IN MYELOFIBROSIS

Chikkappa et al. (28) showed increased numbers of Mk progenitors in the blood and bone marrow of patients with myelofibrosis. Croizat et al. (30) used a plasma clot culture system and detected circulating Mk progenitors in the blood of six of eight patients with PMF but did not detect any in blood from normal individuals. Four of these patients produced Mk colonies in the absence of added PHA-LCM, although addition of PHA-LCM increased the numbers of colonies produced. There may thus be a population of CFU-Mk that is hypersensitive to Mk-CSA and analogous to the Epo hypersensitive erythroid progenitors discussed above. The authors found that the numbers of CFU-Mk increased in one patient as the disease progressed and the patient deteriorated clinically. The cultures became overgrown with Mk so that the colonies could not be counted accurately and these colonies all appeared to be able to grow in the absence of PHA-LCM, i.e., they were presumably derived from the hypersensitive clone. Hibbin et al. (32) also found circulating Mk progenitors in six of 10 patients using a methyl cellulose assay, but they also detected these progenitors in normal peripheral blood (Fig. 1). There was a 167-fold increase in circulating CFU-Mk numbers in patients with MF compared with normals. This increase is much larger than that obtained for the other progenitor cells. They again found no correlation between CFU-Mk numbers and leukocyte or platelet counts, hemoglobin levels, or clinical

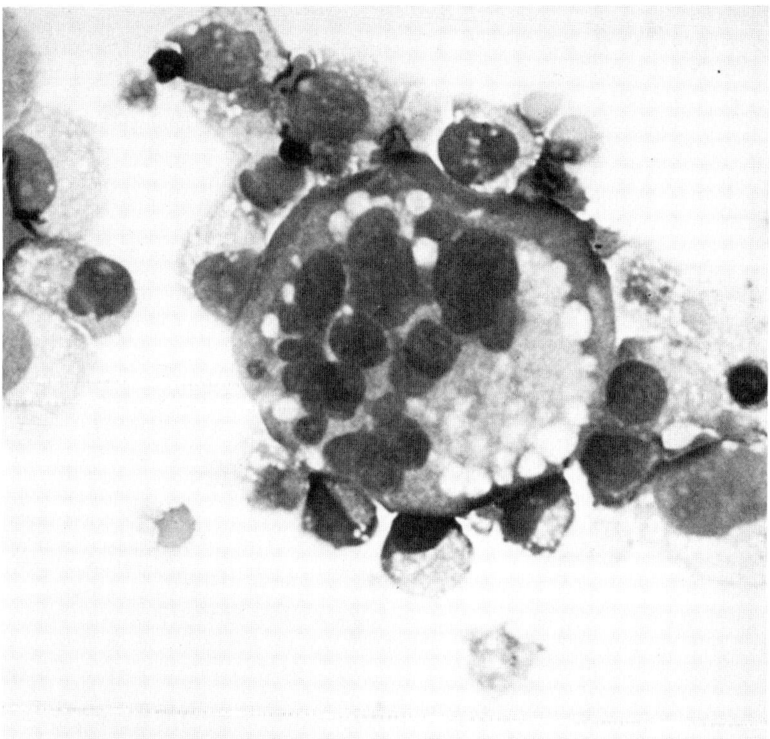

Figure 2 Photograph at light microscopic level of a megakaryocyte cultured in vitro from the blood of a patient with myelofibrosis showing distinctive vacuoles in the cytoplasm and nucleus. May-Grünwald Giemsa stain, 1880X.

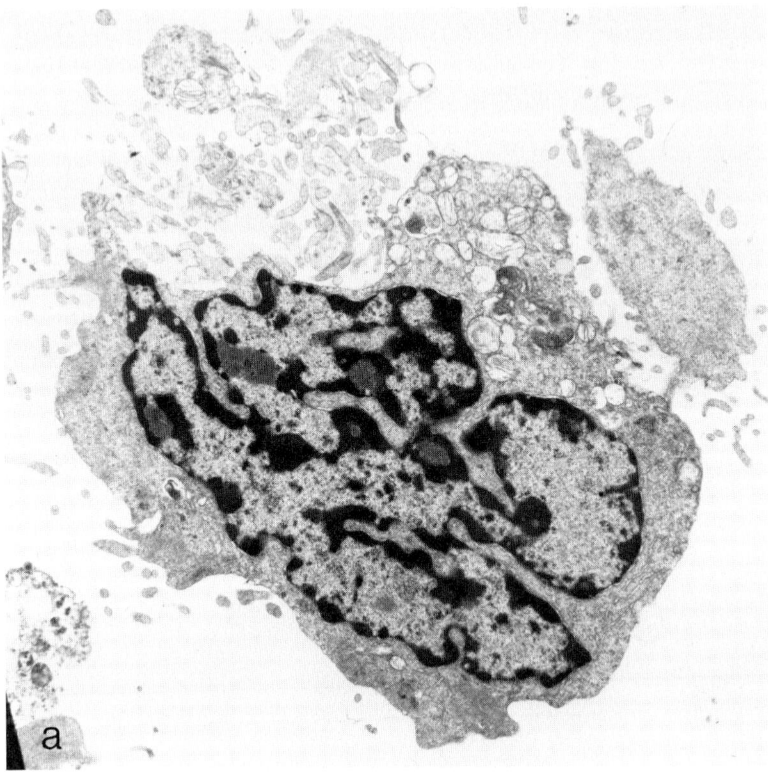

Figure 3 Photographs at electronmicroscope level of megakaryocytes cultured in vitro for 10 days from the blood of a patient with myelofibrosis showing distinctive vacuoles. (a) A large cell with irregular nucleus, few vacuoles, and mitochondria with disrupted cristae. Uranyl acetate and lead nitrate stain, 8,000X.

status of the patient. Some of the cases with the most severe bone marrow fibrosis had no detectable circulating CFU-Mk.

In contrast with the results of Croizat et al. (30), Hibbin et al. (32) found circulating CFU-Mk in two patients with ET; as in PV, their numbers were increased compared with normal in both cases. These latter authors also reported distinctive large vacuoles involving both nucleus and cytoplasm in cultured Mk from every case of PMF and also in cultured Mk from one patient with CGL in megakaryoblastic transformation (Figs. 2 and 3). No such

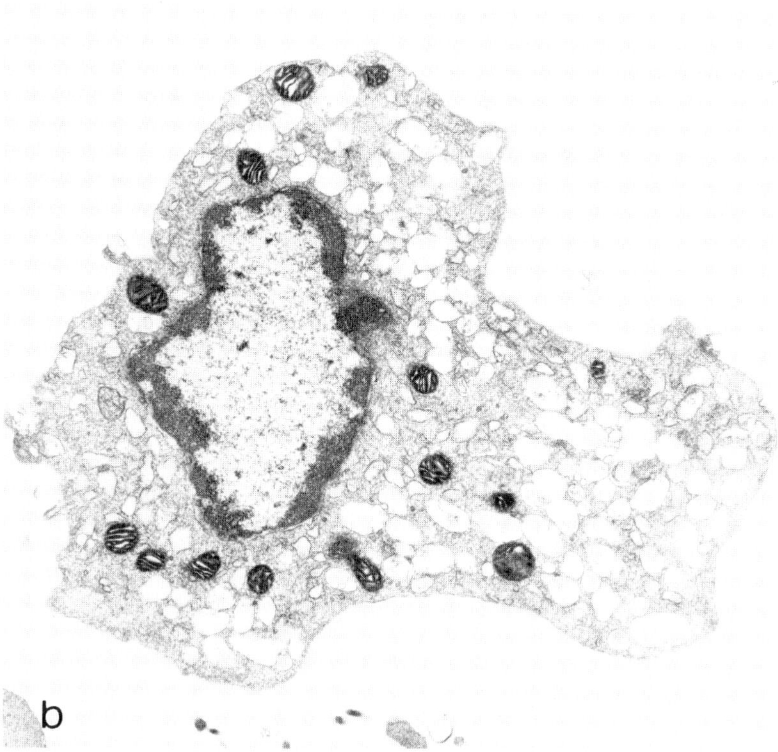

(b) A cell with marked cytoplasmic vacuolation which is not seen in cultures of megakaryocytes from normal bone marrow. Uranyl acetate and lead nitrate stain, 16,000X. (Photographs prepared by Dr. Estela Matutes at the Royal Postgraduate Medical School, London.)

vacuoles were seen in Mk cultured from normal controls or patients with other myeloproliferative disorders. They speculated that this morphological abnormality might reflect a qualitative defect in megakaryocytopoiesis.

MULTIPOTENTIAL PROGENITORS IN MYELOFIBROSIS

Douer et al. (31) showed that two patients with PMF had increased numbers of circulating CFU-GEMM compared with normal individuals. The presence of increased circulating CFU-GEMM was confirmed by Hibbin et al. (32) in six of 10 patients studied (Fig. 1). Both groups found the proportional increase in CFU-GEMM numbers was less than than in CFU-GM or BFU-E numbers; similar results have been obtained with CGL patients (36, 43, 44). The increase in the numbers of earliest multipotential progenitor cells detectable in vitro is further support for the idea that PMF is a pluripotential stem cell disorder.

Fauser and Messner et al. (43) and Ash et al. (46) showed that CFU-GEMM from patients with PV were able to grow in the absence of exogenous Epo, showing that the apparent hypersensitivity previously reported for CFU-E and BFU-E from these patients is also present in more primitive progenitors. The Epo-sensitivity of CFU-GEMM has not yet been studied in patients with PMF. Fauser and Messner (45) also demonstrated increased proliferative activity of CFU-GEMM in PV and suggested that this could be related to the increased formation of blood cells in this disorder. Increased proliferative capacity of CFU-GEMM has also been demonstrated in CGL (44, 47). There is no information on the proliferative status of CFU-GEMM from patients with PMF.

THE ROLE OF THE SPLEEN AS A SITE OF PROGENITOR CELL PRODUCTION IN PMF

Splenomegaly is a regular feature of PMF and the spleen may be a major site of active hemopoiesis in this disorder (2). Goldberg et al. (48) assayed CFU-GM in blood drawn from an arm vein, from the splenic vein, and from the splenic artery in a patient with PMF undergoing splenectomy to reduce excessive transfusion requirements and compared results with those obtained in a patient with Hodgkin's disease undergoing splenectomy during staging laparotomy. The CFU-GM numbers in the PMF patient were higher in the splenic vein blood than in peripheral blood or splenic artery; there was no difference in numbers in the different blood samples from the patient with Hodgkin's disease. These observations suggested that the spleen was an important site of CFU-GM production in PMF.

Koeffler et al. (49) showed that splenic irradiation in PMF caused a significant decrease in circulating CFU-GM, whereas brain irradiation for patients with glioma as controls had no effect on circulating CFU-GM numbers. The authors could detect no radiation-induced humoral inhibitor of granulopoiesis and the PMF patients did not have increased CFU-GM radiosensitivity; they concluded that the irradiation induced the granulocytopenia in PMF by destroying proliferating precursors in the spleen. Kirschner et al. (33) assayed CFU-GM in the splenic vein and artery in two patients with PMF; in both cases, the numbers in the splenic vein were higher than in splenic artery or peripheral blood. In one patient, the circulating CFU-GM fell and remained low after splenectomy, whereas in the other patient the numbers were not significantly lower 5 months later. The authors suggested therefore that in the first patient the spleen was virtually the only source of CFU-GM production whereas in the second there must have been some contribution from residual bone marrow and/or liver.

Partanen et al. (29) found no differences in circulating CFU-GM, CFU-E, or BFU-E numbers between splenectomized and nonsplenectomized patients. In contrast, Wang et al. (34) suggested that the increased circulating CFU-GM numbers found in patients with PMF compared with patients with SMF could be explained by the increased splenomegaly in the patients with PMF. Hibbin et al. (32) found no significant difference in circulating CFU-GM numbers between splenectomized and nonsplenectomized patients, although they found no circulating BFU-E, CFU-Mk, or CFU-GEMM in splenectomized patients. There was no explanation for the difference between results for CFU-GM and those of the other progenitor cells. Studies on the same patient before and after splenectomy will be necessary to elucidate the effects on all circulating progenitor cell numbers.

In summary, it appears that the spleen, at least for some patients with PMF, may play a major role in hemopoiesis. Splenectomy for these patients would be expected to reduce the numbers of circulating progenitors. In other patients, however, significant hematopoiesis must also take place at other extramedullary sites and thus splenectomy would have little or no effect on circulating progenitor cell numbers.

EFFECTS OF PROSTAGLANDIN E_1 (PGE_1) ON COLONY FORMATION IN PMF

CFU-GM from normal individuals are dependent on CSA for their growth in vitro; conversely PGE_1 inhibits the growth of CFU-GM in a dose-dependent manner, possibly by competition with CSA (50, 51).

Taetle and co-authors (52, 53) showed that CFU-GM grown from patients with CGL were inhibited by PGE_1 in the absence of exogenous CSA but that addition of increasing amounts of CSA offset this inhibition. They showed that CSA was able to decrease the PGE_1 inhibition in these patients, even at CSA concentrations that were unable to overcome the inhibition in normal individuals. They suggested that this may be one way in which CGL progenitors express a proliferative advantage over their normal counterparts. PGE_1 and CSA each regulate the production of the other so it is equally possible that the abnormal PGE_1 and CSA competition found in CGL patients is merely an exaggeration of a normal regulatory mechanism.

Taetle et al. (53) also tested the effects of PGE_1 on CFU-GM from patients with PMF and found that the dose-response curves showed great variability; some patients showed the normal inhibition and others stimulation. They fractionated the cells on low-density Ficoll gradients and found two populations of cells, one showing normal inhibition by PGE_1 and the other, which did not respond normally. They could not explain the PGE_1-mediated increase in CFU-GM numbers but showed that it was not due to release of CSA or other enhancers from the adherent cells. They suggested that PGE_1 might be converted to another prostaglandin, e.g., $PGF_{2\alpha}$, which has a stimulatory effect on CFU-GM. This conversion occurs in mice (54).

Aglietta et al. (55) also tested the effects of PGE_1 on circulating CFU-GM in eight patients with PMF and found their growth uninhibited by concentrations of PGE_1 in the range 10^{10} to 10^6 *M*: normal CFU-GM were inhibited at these concentrations. Pelus et al. (56) suggested that a subpopulation of CFU-GM, the monocyte/macrophage progenitors, were more sensitive to PGE_1 than the granulocyte progenitors. Taetle et al. (53) and Aglietta et al. (55) showed, however, that there were macrophages in the colonies produced in the presence of PGE_1. These groups both suggested that the PGE_1-mediated effects could be one method by which the abnormal myeloid progenitors might gain a proliferative advantage and contribute to the increased myelopoiesis seen in PMF.

HEMOPOIETIC PROGENITOR CELLS AND THE PATHOPHYSIOLOGY OF PMF

The Stem Cell Defects

Croizat et al. (30) assayed CFU-GM, BFU-E, and CFU-Mk in peripheral blood samples from patients with PV, ET, and PMF. They concluded that there were abnormalities in the different lineages, expressed at the level of the circulating committed progenitor cells, that were characteristic for the different myeloproliferative disorders. Their results differed in some instances from those obtained by other groups (29, 32). On the basis of their results, however, Croizat et al. (30) postulated that two lesions might occur in the development of the different myeloproliferative disorders. They envisaged an initial regulatory defect in a pluripotential stem cell, which would confer a growth advantage on these cells and allow a "pathological" clone to emerge. They then suggested that a second lesion could occur within this clone that would differ in the different myeloproliferative disorders, e.g., the lesion in PMF would lead specifically to abnormal populations of circulating CFU-GM and CFU-Mk. Fialkow et al. (57) proposed a similar multistep mechanism for the pathogenesis of CGL. Other workers also demonstrated elevated numbers of one or both of these progenitors in all myeloproliferative disorders (29, 32, 39).

Platelet-Derived Growth Factor (PDGF)

Human platelets contain a growth factor, PDGF, which promotes the growth in vitro of fibroblasts (58, 59), of glial (60) and of smooth muscle cells (61). PDGF is a heat-stable polypeptide. Each platelet contains about 1000 molecules of PDGF stored in alpha granules (62) and PDGF is released into the serum during the clotting process. Receptors for PDGF have been found on diploid human fibroblasts (63). Pledger et al. (64) showed that PDGF in serum was needed to stimulate resting (G_0) fibroblasts to enter cell cycle (G_1). Recently, two groups (65, 66) independently showed that the amino acid sequence of part of the PDGF molecule (67) is almost identical to that of the putative transforming protein (p28-*sis*) of the cellular oncogene c-*sis*.

Michalevicz et al. (68) showed that PDGF promoted proliferation of CFU-GEMM and Francis et al. (69) suggested that aberrant expression of c-*sis* in CGL (due to translocation of c-*sis* from the Philadelphia chromosome, chromosome 22q−, to chromosome 9q+) might account for the increased CFU-GEMM and hence the excess proliferation of other progenitor cells in this disease. The observation however that c-*sis* is normally located at a considerable distance from the breakpoint on the Philadelphia chromosome, and thus presumably at some distance from possible new controlling genes on chromosome 9q+, accords poorly with this hypothesis (70).

Role of Megakaryocytes and PDGF in PMF

Groopman (71) showed that abnormal platelets from patients with myeloproliferative disorders released PDGF, which stimulated the proliferation of fibroblasts and reticulin synthesis. He suggested that an acquired defect in the storage of PDGF in the alpha granules might lead to leakage of PDGF which in turn could stimulate fibroblast proliferation. The suggestion could also explain why not all disorders involving increased megakaryocytopoiesis result in marrow fibrosis (e.g., secondary thrombocytosis); the platelets in such disorders may not be not defective.

Castro-Malaspina et al. (72) separated human bone marrow cells in density gradients and tested the growth promoting activities of homogenates of the different fractions on normal human fibroblasts. They found maximum growth promotion in homogenates of the megakaryocyte- and the platelet-enriched fractions. The dose-response curves for these two fractions were parallel, suggesting the presence of analogous growth factors derived from megakaryocytes (MkDGF) and platelets (PDGF). These results led them to postulate a mechanism for the development of PMF (73). They suggested that the defective Mk maturation, which is recognized in PMF (2, 74, 75), results in the death of many Mk in the bone marrow. Mk and platelet-derived components, particularly MkDGF and platelet factor 4, then escape into the intracellular spaces. High concentrations of MkDGF stimulate the fibroblasts to proliferate and produce collagen. The excess collagen would normally be degraded by collagenases but platelet factor 4, now present in excess, inhibits collagenase activity (76). It is thus the combination of increased fibroblast proliferation and collagen production with decreased collagen degradation that leads to the fibrosis.

They, like Groopman, suggested that excessive ineffective megakaryocytopoiesis must be important in PMF because expanded Mk numbers alone do not necessarily result in myelofibrosis. This hypothesis can also account for the fibrosis observed in acute megakaryoblastic leukemia, since Rabellino et al. (77) found that synthesis of products found in mature Mk begins at an early age. The increased death of megakaryoblasts could result in the presence of abnormal amounts of Mk-derived products in the bone marrow milieu.

Croizat et al. (30) reported increased circulating CFU-Mk numbers in patients with PMF; these CFU-Mk were insensitive to normal Mk regulators in vitro. In one patient in an advanced phase of his disease, the majority of the cultured Mk were independent of (or highly sensitive to) added stimulator and therefore presumably derived from an abnormal clone. Hibbin et al. (32) also observed an increase in circulating CFU-Mk numbers from patients with PMF; these Mk had a morphological abnormality that could have been due at least in part to loss of alpha granules. These observations provide further support for the Castro-Malaspina and Moore model, since the expanded population of abnormal Mk progenitors in the circulation may reflect the same defect in the Mk population in the marrow.

Bianchi-Scarra et al. (78) showed that there was increased fibroblast proliferation in bone marrow from patients with increased marrow Mk numbers or increased blood platelet counts, regardless of the underlying disorders, which suggested a quantitative mechanism alone for development of Mk without the need for a qualitative defect in the Mk or platelets. The recent finding that PDGF has homology with p28-*sis*, the transforming protein of the c-*sis* oncogene, suggests that c-*sis* may be abnormally expressed in these patients. All of these reports of Mk- and PDGF-mediated fibrosis provide more evidence for a clonal defect in a hematopoietic progenitor in PMF and show the importance of characterizing the hematopoietic progenitors in this disease.

VITAMIN D AND MYELOFIBROSIS

There is both clinical and laboratory evidence that vitamin D may be involved in the regulation of collagen deposition in the marrow. Cooperberg and Singer (79) described an infant with rickets and increased fibrous tissue in the marrow. After vitamin D treatment, the fibrosis regressed and the spleen returned to its normal size. More recently Yetgin and Ozsoylu (80) described a group of 11 patients with severe nutritional rickets, extramedullary hemopoiesis, and anemia with red cell morphology typical of PMF. Six of the patients had vitamin D administered. They showed hematopoietic improvement, and their liver and spleen sizes decreased.

McCarthy et al. (81) showed that 1,25-dihydroxyvitamin D_3 [1,25-$(OH)_2$ D_3], the most active metabolite of vitamin D_3, inhibited the proliferation of CFU-Mk from both normal marrow and PMF blood in a dose-dependent manner. McCarthy et al. (82) suggested that 1,25-$(OH)_2$ D_3 may play a role in control of bone marrow collagen deposition (Fig. 4): 1,25-$(OH)_2$ D_3

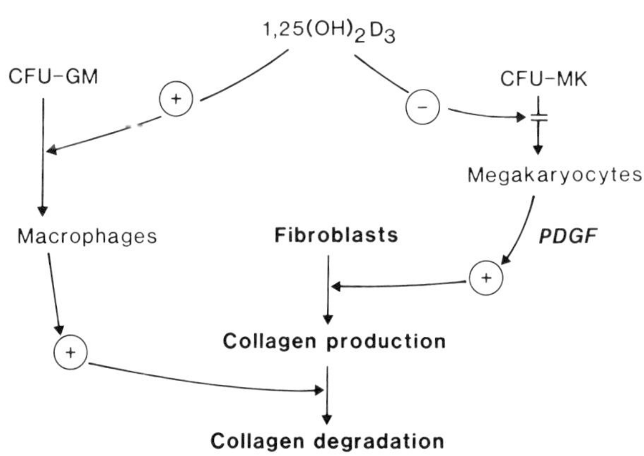

Figure 4 Schematic representation of the possible effects of vitamin D_3 on megakaryocyte proliferation and collagen deposition and degradation in the bone marrow. (+) Indicates stimulation; (-) indicates inhibition. PDGF = platelet-derived growth factor. [Reproduced from McCarthy et al. (Ref. 82) with permission of the publishers.]

inhibits Mk proliferation and this in turn might reduce Mk-dependent fibroblast proliferation and collagen synthesis. The 1,25-$(OH)_2$ D_3 may also act directly by inhibiting collagen synthesis. Fibrous tissue may be normally degraded by collagenases produced by monocytes and macrophages, and the production of these cells is increased at least in vitro by 1,25-$(OH)_2$ D_3 (83, 84). The presence of 1,25-$(OH)_2$ D_3 therefore may antagonize collagen synthesis, whereas a deficiency would allow abnormal accumulation of collagen in the marrow and hence myelofibrosis.

CONCLUSIONS

The various hemopoietic progenitor cells are numerically increased in the circulation of patients with primary myelofibrosis; this and chromosomal evidence suggest that PMF is due to a primary defect in a pluripotential hematopoietic stem cell. A proportion of these progenitor cells can proliferate and form colonies in vitro in the absence of the stimulatory factors normally required for colony formation. There may thus coexist two (or more) populations, one with normal dependence on exogenous factors and the other hypersensitive and thereby responsive to minute quantities of stimulatory factors (or indeed capable of proliferation in their absence); the latter might have some long-term proliferative advantage over the former.

In PMF the Mk progenitor compartment is enlarged to a greater extent than other progenitor compartments. Morphological abnormalities are found in the Mk that develop in liquid culture and in semisolid media. PMF may be due to an increased but ineffective megakaryocytopoiesis in the bone marrow which causes excessive amounts of PDGF and platelet factor 4 to be released into intercellular spaces and consequently marrow fibrosis.

The selective inhibition of CFU-Mk proliferation by the active metabolite of vitamin D_3 and the finding that some infants with rickets have blood and marrow pictures resembling myelofibrosis may mean that vitamin D plays a role in control of collagen deposition in the normal marrow.

REFERENCES

1. Dameshek, W. (1951). Some speculations on the myeloproliferative syndromes. *Blood 6*: 372–376.
2. Ward, H. P., and Block, M. H. (1971). The natural history of agnogenic myeloid metaplasia (AMM) and a critical evaluation of its relationship with the myeloproliferative syndrome. *Medicine 50*: 357–420.
3. Van Slyck, E. J., Weiss, L., and Dully, M. (1970). Chromosomal evidence

for the secondary role of bone marrow fibroblast proliferation in acute myelofibrosis. *Blood 36*: 729–735.

4. Khan, A., Bernard, J. F., Cottreau, D., Marie, J., Bowin, P., and Abrami, G. (1975). A deficient G6PD variant with hemizygous expression in blood cells of a woman with primary myelofibrosis. *Humangenetik 30*: 41–46.
5. Jacobson, R. J., Salo, A., and Fialkow, P. J. (1978). Agnogenic myeloid metaplasia: a clonal proliferation of hemopoietic stem cells with secondary myelofibrosis. *Blood 51*: 189–194.
6. Rappeport, J., Parkman, R., Belli, J., Levey, R., Rosen, F., and Nathan, D. (1978). Reversibility of myelofibrosis (MF) after bone marrow transplantation (abstract). *Blood 52* (suppl. 1): 598.

6a. Smith, J. W., Shulman, H. M., Thomas, E. D., Fefer, A., and Buckner, C. D. (1981). Bone marrow transplantation for acute myelosclerosis. *Cancer 48*: 2198–2203.

7. Wolf, J. L., Spruce, W. E., Bearman, R. M., Forman, S. J. Scott, E. P., Fahey, J. L., Fabstein, M. J., Rappaport, H., and Blume, K. G. (1982). Reversal of acute ('malignant') myelosclerosis by allogeneic bone marrow transplantation. *Blood 59*: 191–193.
8. Oblon, D. J., Elfenbein, G. J., Braylan, R. C., Jones, J., and Weiner, R. J. (1983). The reversal of myelofibrosis associated with chronic myelogenous leukemia after bone marrow transplantation. *Exp. Hematol. 11*: 681–685.
9. Pike, B., and Robinson, W. A. (1970). Human bone marrow culture in agar gel. *J. Cell Physiol. 76*: 77–84.
10. Bradley, T. R., and Metcalf, D. (1966). The growth of mouse bone marrow cells in-vitro. *Aust. J. Exp. Biol. Med. Sci. 44*: 287–300.
11. Metcalf, D., Parker, J., Chester, H. M., and Kincade, P. W. (1974). Formation of eosinophil-like granulocytic colonies by mouse bone marrow cells in-vitro. *J. Cell Physiol. 84*: 275–290.
12. Tepperman, A. D., Curtis, J. E., and McCulloch, E. A. (1974). Erythropoietic colonies in cultures of human marrow. *Blood 44*: 659–669.
13. Stephenson, J. R., Axelrad, A. A., McLeod, D. L., and Shreeve, M. M. (1971). Induction of colonies of hemoglobin-synthesizing cells by erythropoietin in-vitro. *Proc. Natl. Acad. Sci. USA 68*: 1542–1546.
14. McLeod, D. L., Shreeve, M. M., and Axelrad, A. A. (1974). Improved plasma culture system for production of erythrocytic colonies in-vitro: Quantitative assay method for CFU-E. *Blood 44*: 517–534.
15. Iscove, N. N., Sieber, F., and Winterhalter, K. H. (1974). Erythroid colony formation in cultures of mouse and human bone marrow. Analysis of the requirement for erythropoietin by gel filtration and affinity chromatography on agarose-concanavalin A. *J. Cell Physiol. 83*: 309–320.

16. Bonsdorff, E., and Jalavisto, E. (1948). A humoral mechanism in anoxic erythrocytosis. *Acta Haem. Scand. 16*: 150–170.
17. Clarke, B. J., and Housman, D. (1977). Characterisation of an erythroid precursor cell of high proliferative capacity in normal human peripheral blood. *Proc. Natl. Acad. Sci. USA 74*: 1105–1109.
18. Vainchenker, W., Guichard, J., and Breton-Gorius, J. (1979). Growth of human megakaryocyte colonies in culture from fetal, neonatal and adult peripheral blood cells. Ultrastructural analysis. *Blood Cells 5*: 25–42.
19. Vainchenker, W., Bouguet, J., Guichard, J., and Breton-Gorius, J. (1979). Megakaryocyte colony formation from human bone marrow precursors. *Blood 54*: 940–945.
20. Messner H. A., Jamal, N., and Izaguirre, C. A. (1982). Growth of large megakaryocyte colonies from normal human bone marrow. *J. Cell Physiol.* (suppl. 1): 45–51.
21. Vainchenker, W., Chapman, J., Deschamps, J. F., Vinci, G., Bouguet, J., Titeux, M., and Breton-Gorius, J. (1982). Normal human serum contains a factor(s) capable of inhibiting megakaryocyte colony formation. *Exp. Hematol. 10*: 650–660.
22. Williams, N., and Levine, R. F. (1982). The origin, development and regulation of megakaryocytes. *Br. J. Haematol. 52*: 173–180.
23. Fauser, A. A., and Messner, H. A. (1979). Identification of megakaryocytes, macrophages and eosinophils in colonies of human bone marrow containing neutrophilic granulocytes and erythroblasts. *Blood 53*: 1023–1027.
24. Ash, R. C., Detrick, R. A., and Zanjani, E. D. (1981). Studies of human pluripotential hemopoietic stem cells (CFU-GEMM) in-vitro. *Blood 58*: 309–316.
25. Chervenick, P. A. (1973). Increase in circulating stem cells in patients with myelofibrosis. *Blood 41*: 67–71.
26. Ohl, S., Carsten, A. L., Chanana, A. D., Chikkappa, G., and Cronkite, E. P. (1976). Increased erythrocytic and neutrophilic progenitors in myelofibrosis with myeloid metaplasia. *Eur. J. Cancer 12*: 131–135.
27. Goldman, J. M., Seitanides, B., Ruutu, T., and Th'ng, K. H. (1978). Granulocyte-committed progenitor cells in the blood of patients with myelosclerosis. *Scand. J. Haematol. 21*: 318–322.
28. Chikkappa, G., Carsten, A. L., Chanana, A. D., Chandra, P., and Cronkite, E. P. (1978). Increased granulocytic, erythrocytic and megakaryocytic progenitors in myelofibrosis with myeloid metaplasia. *Am. J. Hematol. 4*: 121–131.
29. Partanen, S., Ruutu, T., and Vuopio, P. (1982). Circulating haematopoietic progenitors in myelofibrosis. *Scand. J. Haematol. 29*: 325–330.
30. Croizat, H., Amato, D., McLeod, D. L., Eskinazi, D., and Axelrad, A. A. (1983). Differences among myeloproliferative disorders in the behaviour of their restricted progenitor cells in culture. *Blood 62*: 578–584.

31. Douer, D., Fabian, I., and Cline, M. J. (1983). Circulating pluripotent haemopoietic cells in patients with myeloproliferative disorders. *Br. J. Haematol. 54*: 373–381.
32. Hibbin, J. A., Njoku, O. S., Matutes, E., Lewis, S. M., and Goldman, J. M. (1984). Myeloid progenitor cells in the circulation of patients with myelofibrosis and other myeloproliferative disorders. *Br. J. Haematol. 57*: 495–504.
33. Kirschner, J. J., Goldberg, J., and Landaw, S. A. (1980). The spleen as a site of colony forming cell production in myelofibrosis. *Proc. Soc. Exp. Biol. Med. 165*: 279–282.
34. Wang, J. C., Cheung, C. P., Ahmed, F., Steier, W., and Tobin, M. S. (1983). Circulating granulocyte and macrophage progenitor cells in primary and secondary myelofibrosis. *Br. J. Haematol. 54*: 301–308.
35. Lacombe, C., Casadevall, N., and Varet, B. (1980). Polycythaemia vera: In-vitro studies of circulating erythroid progenitors. *Br. J. Haematol. 44*: 189–199.
36. Goldman, J. M., Shiota, F., Th'ng, K. H., and Orchard, K. H. (1980). Circulating granulocytic and erythroid progenitor cells in chronic granulocytic leukaemia. *Br. J. Haematol. 46*: 7–13.
37. Prchal, J. F., Axelrad, A. A., and Crookston, J. H. (1974). Erythroid colony formation in plasma culture from cells of peripheral blood in myeloproliferative disorders (abstract). *Blood 44*: 912a.
38. Lutton, J. D., and Levere, R. D. (1984). Endogenous erythroid colony formation by peripheral blood mononuclear cells from patients with myelofibrosis and polycythaemia vera. *Acta Haematol. 62*: 94–99.
39. Kornberg, A., Fibach, E., Treves, A., Goldfarb, A., and Rachmilewitz, E. A. (1982). Circulating erythroid progenitors in patients with 'spent' polycythaemia vera and myelofibrosis with myeloid metaplasia. *Br. J. Haematol. 52*: 573–578.
40. Prchal, J. F., and Axelrad, A. A. (1974). Bone marrow responses in polycythemia vera. *New Engl. J. Med. 290*: 1382.
41. Zanjani, E. D., Lutton, J. D., Hoffman, R., and Wasserman, L. R. (1977). Erythroid colony formation by polycythemia vera bone marrow in-vitro. *J. Clin. Invest. 59*: 841–848.
42. Casadevall, N., Vainchenker, W., Lacombe, C., Vinci, G., Chapman, J., Breton-Gorius, J., and Varet, B. (1982). Erthyroid progenitors in polycythemia vera: demonstration of their hypersensitivity to erythropoietin using serum-free cultures. *Blood 59*: 447–451.
43. Goldman, J. M., Th'ng, K. H., and Lowenthal, R. M. (1974). In-vitro colony forming cells and colony stimulating factor in chronic granulocytic leukaemia. *Br. J. Cancer 30*: 1–12.
44. Hibbin, J. A., McCarthy, D. M., and Goldman, J. M. (1983). Antigenic expression and proliferative status of multilineage myeloid progenitor cells (CFU-GEMM) in normal individuals and patients with chronic granulocytic leukaemia. *Scand. J. Haematol. 31*: 454–460.

45. Fauser, A. A., and Messner, H. A. (1981). Pluripotent hemopoietic progenitors (CFU-GEMM) in polycythemia vera: Analysis of erythropoietin requirement and proliferative activity. *Blood 58*: 1224–1227.
46. Ash, R. C., Detrick, R. A., and Zanjani, E. D. (1982). In-vitro studies of human pluripotential hemopoietic progenitors in polycythemia vera: Direct evidence of stem cell involvement. *J. Clin. Invest. 69*: 1112–1118.
47. Lepine, J., and Messner, H. A. (1983). Pluripotent hemopoietic progenitors (CFU-GEMM) in chronic myelogenous leukemia. *Int. J. Cell Cloning 1*: 230–239.
48. Goldberg, J., Tice, D., Nelson, D., Landaw, S. A., and Gottlieb, A. J. (1977). The spleen as a site of colony forming cell production in primary myelofibrosis. *Blood 50* (suppl. 1): 148 (abstract 221).
49. Koeffler, H. P., Cline, M. J., and Golde, D. W. (1979). Splenic irradiation in myelofibrosis: effect on circulating myeloid progenitor cells. *Br. J. Haematol. 43*: 69–77.
50. Kurland, J. I., and Moore, M. A. S. (1977). Modulation of hemopoiesis by prostaglandins. *Exp. Hematol. 5*: 357–373.
51. Kurland, J. I., Broxmeyer, H. E., Pelus, L. M., Bockman, R. S., and Moore, M. A. S. (1978). Role of monocyte/macrophage-derived colony-stimulating factor and prostaglandin E in the positive and negative feedback control of myeloid stem cell proliferation. *Blood 52*: 388–407.
52. Taetle, R., and Koessler, A. (1980). Effects of cyclic nucleotides and prostaglandins on normal and abnormal human myeloid progenitor proliferation. *Cancer Res. 40*: 1223–1229.
53. Taetle, R., Guittard, J. P., and Mendelsohn, I. (1980). Abnormal modulation of granulocyte/macrophage progenitor proliferation by prostaglandin E in chronic myeloproliferative disorders. *Exp. Hematol. 8*: 1190–1201.
54. Ziboh, V. A., Lord, J. I., Blick, G., Kursunuglu, I., Poitier, J., and Yunis, A. (1977). Alteration of prostaglandin biosynthesis in rat chloroleukemic tumor. *Cancer Res. 37*: 3974–3980.
55. Aglietta, M., Piacibello, W., and Gavosto, F. (1981). Myelofibrosis and prostaglandins: effect of prostaglandin E1 on colony forming cells (CFU-GM). *Br. J. Haematol. 48*: 167–169.
56. Pelus, L. M., Broxmeyer, H. E., Kurland, J. I., and Moore, M. A. S. (1979). Regulation of macrophage and granulocyte proliferation. Specificities of prostaglandin E and lactoferrin. *J. Exp. Med. 150*: 277–292.
57. Fialkow, P. J., Martin, P. J., Najfeld, V., Penfold, G. K., Jacobson, R. J., and Hansen, J. A. (1981). Evidence for a multistep pathogenesis of chronic myelogenous leukemia. *Blood 58*: 158–163.
58. Kohler, N., and Lipton, A. (1974). Platelets as a source of a fibroblast growth promoting activity. *Exp. Cell Res. 87*: 297–301.
59. Antoniades, H. N., and Scher, C. D. (1977). Radioimmunoassay of a

human serum growth factor for Balb/c-3T3 cells. Derivation from platelets. *Proc. Natl. Acad. Sci. USA 74*: 1973–1977.
60. Westermark, B., and Wasteson, A. (1976). A platelet factor stimulating human normal glial cells. *Exp. Cell Res. 98*: 170–174.
61. Ross, R. J., Glomset, J., Kariya, B., and Harker, L. (1974). A platelet-dependent serum factor that stimulates the proliferation of arterial smooth muscle cells in-vitro. *Proc. Natl. Acad. Sci. USA 71*: 1207–1210.
62. Ross, R., and Vogel, A. (1978). The platelet-derived growth factor. *Cell 14*: 203–210.
63. Stiles, C. D. (1983). The molecular biology of platelet-derived growth factor. *Cell 33*: 653–655.
64. Pledger, W. J., Stiles, C. D., Antoniades, H. N., and Scher, C. D. (1978). An ordered sequence of events is required before Balb/c-3T3 cells become committed to DNA synthesis. *Proc. Natl. Acad. Sci. USA 75*: 2839–2843.
65. Waterfield, M. D., Scrace, G. T., Whittle, N., Stroobant, P., Johnsson, A., Wasteson, B., Westermark, A., Heldin, C-H., Huang, J. S., and Devel, T. F. (1983). Platelet-derived growth factor is structurally related to the putative transforming protein $p28^{sis}$ of simian sarcoma virus. *Nature 304*: 35–39.
66. Doolittle, R. F., Hunkapiller, M. W., Hood, L. E., Devare, S. G., Robbins, K. C., Aaronson, S. A., and Antoniades, H. N. (1983). Simian sarcoma virus *onc* gene v-*sis* is derived from the gene (or genes) encoding a platelet-derived growth factor. *Science 221*: 275–176.
67. Devarre, S. G., Reddy, E. P., Law, J. D., Robbins, K. C., Aaronson, S. A., and Antoniades, H. N. (1983). Nucleotide sequence of the simian sarcoma virus genome: demonstration that its acquired cellular sequences encode the transforming gene product $p28^{sis}$. *Proc. Natl. Acad. Sci. USA 80*: 731–735.
68. Michalevicz, R., Francis, G. E., Price, G., and Hoffbrand, A. V. (1984). Platelet-derived growth factor promotes proliferation of CFU-GEMM in-vitro. *Blood 62* (suppl. 1): 139a (abstract).
69. Francis, G. E., Michalevicz, R., and Wickramasinghe, R. G. (1983). Chronic myeloid leukemia and the Philadelphia translocation: Do the c-*sis* oncogene and platelet-derived growth factor provide the link? *Leuk. Res. 7*: 817–820.
70. Bartram, C. R., De Klein, A., Hagemeijer, A., Grosveld, G., Heisterkamp, N., and Groffen, J. (1984). Localization of human c-sis oncogene in Ph^1-positive and Ph^1-negative chronic myelocytic leukemia by in-situ hybridization. *Blood 63*: 223–225.
71. Groopman, J. E. (1980). The pathogenesis of myelofibrosis in myeloproliferative disorders. *Ann. Intern. Med. 92*: 857–858.
72. Castro-Malaspina, H., Rabellino, E. M., Yen, A., Nachman, R. L., and

Moore, M. A. S. (1981). Human megakaryocyte stimulation of proliferation of bone marrow fibroblasts. *Blood 57*: 781–787.
73. Castro-Malaspina, H., and Moore, M. A. S. (1982). Pathophysiological mechanisms operating in the development of myelofibrosis: role of megakaryocytes. *Nouv. Rev. Franc. Hemat. 24*: 221–226.
74. Kass, L. (1979). Agnogenic myeloid metaplasia. In *Bone Marrow Interpretation.* Edited by L. Kass, Philadelphia, J. B. Lippincott Co, pp. 224–227.
75. Thiele, J., Ballard, A-Ch., Georgii, A., and Vykoupil, K. F. (1977). Chronic megakaryocytic-granulocytic myelosis. An electron microscopy study. I. Megakaryocytes and thrombocytes. *Virch. Arch. (Pathol. Anat.) 313*: 191–211.
76. Hiti-Harper, J., Wohl, H., and Harper, E. (1978). Platelet factor 4: An inhibitor of collagenase. *Science 199*: 991–992.
77. Rabellino, E. M., Levene, R. B., Leung, L. L. K., and Nachman, R. L. (1981). Human megakaryocytes. II. Expression of platelet proteins in early marrow megakaryocytes. *J. Exp. Med. 154*: 88–100.
78. Bianchi-Scarra, G. L., Barresi, R., Ajmar, F., Garre, C., Ravazzolo, R., and Sessarego, M. (1983). Fibroblastoid colony-forming cells in myeloproliferative disorders. *Acta Haematol. 70*: 349–356.
79. Cooperberg, A. A., and Singer, O. P. (1966). Reversible myelofibrosis due to vitamin D deficiency rickets. *Canad. Med. Ass. J. 94*: 392–395.
80. Yetgin, and Ozsoylu, S. (1982). Myeloid metaplasia in vitamin D deficiency rickets. *Scand. J. Haematol. 28*: 180–185.
81. McCarthy, D. M., Hibbin, J. A., Daniel, C. P., and Goldman, J. M. (1984). Inhibition of proliferation of megakaryocyte progenitor cells in-vitro by 1,25-dihydroxyvitamin D_3. *Br. J. Haematol. 56*: 670–671 (abstract).
82. McCarthy, D. M., Hibbin, J. A., and Goldman, J. M. (1984). A role for 1,25-dihydroxyvitamin D_3 in control of bone marrow collagen deposition? *Lancet i*: 78–80.
83. McCarthy, D. M., San Miguel, J. F., Freake, H. C., Green, P. M., Zola, H., Catovsky, D., Goldman, J. M. (1983). 1,25-Dihydroxyvitamin D_3 inhibits proliferation of human promyelocytic leukemia HL60 cells and induces monocyte-macrophage differentiation in HL60 and normal bone marrow cells. *Leuk. Res. 7*: 51–55.
84. Moore, M. A. S., Gabrilove, J., and Sheridan, A. P. (1983). Induction of myeloid leukemic cell differentiation by endogenous cytokines or vitamin analogues. In *Leukemia Research, Advances in Cell Biology and Treatment.* Edited by S. B. Murphy and J. R. Gilbert. New York, Elsevier, pp. 32–51.

6

Ferrokinetics and Erythrokinetic Studies in Myelofibrosis

AUGUSTIN FERRANT
University of Louvain Medical School, Brussels, Belgium

INTRODUCTION

Chronic primary myelofibrosis (PMF) is a disease in which extramedullary erythropoiesis is associated with a variable degree of bone marrow fibrosis and, usually, anemia. Knowledge of both the pathophysiology of anemia and the site of erythropoiesis is of value in PMF because the amount of extramedullary erythropoiesis and the efficiency of erythropoiesis may differ markedly from one patient to another. Radionuclide studies with iron- and chromium-labeled red cells have provided a valuable means of assessing the degree of anemia and localizing the sites of active erythropoiesis. The information thus provided may be useful to confirm a diagnosis of PMF, to evaluate the prognosis, and to make therapeutic decisions.

METHODS

Red Cell Survival

The method most widely used for the determination of the mean red cell survival uses ^{51}Cr-labeled autologous red cells (1). The normal mean red cell life span is about 110 days. Surface radioactivity measurements over liver and spleen after infusion of ^{51}Cr-labeled red cells can provide information on the importance of red cell destruction in these organs (2).

Ferrokinetics

Ferrokinetics with ^{59}Fe-transferrin are most useful for measuring total hemoglobin synthesis and for differentiating between the components of hemoglobin synthesis that will be incorporated into circulating red cells from those that will not be so incorporated (3).

The measurements include plasma iron half-life, plasma iron turnover, and percentage of ^{59}Fe in the red cells 14 days after injection of ^{59}Fe-transferrin (red cell utilization). The normal values are 60–120 min for the plasma iron half-life, 100–150 μmol/liter of blood/day for the plasma iron turnover and ±80% for the red cell utilization. The plasma iron disappearance and red cell utilization can be analyzed further to obtain the effective red cell iron turnover, which is a measurement of the effective erythropoiesis. The ineffective iron turnover, extravascular iron turnover, and tissue iron turnover can also be measured (4).

Surface counting demonstrates the sites of radioactive iron uptake. Transferrin-iron uptake in the marrow or the spleen implies the presence of erythropoiesis at these sites. Bone marrow scanning identifies sites of uptake more clearly than does surface counting. ^{59}Fe can be used for this purpose, but its long half-life (45.7 days) and the high energy of its gamma rays (1.1 and 1.3 MeV) are not optimal for scanning. Cyclotron-produced ^{52}Fe has a 8.2 half-life and is a positron emitter (5). Its physical characteristics are more suitable for bone marrow scanning than ^{59}Fe. Bone-marrow scanning with ^{52}Fe is performed when most of the radioiron has left the circulation, i.e., between 2 and 24 hr after injection. Quantitative scanning allows the measurement of the fraction of the injection iron in the skeleton, the liver and the spleen (6, 7).

$^{111}InCl_3$ has also been used for bone marrow scanning, but the distribution of this radionuclide does not reflect precisely the sites or the amount of erythropoiesis (8).

Measurement of the Blood Volumes

Splenomegaly is associated with an increased splenic red cell pool (9) and an enlarged plasma volume (10). In such cases, the hemoglobin concentration in the peripheral blood does not reflect the magnitude of the red cell mass. In patients with an enlarged spleen, measurement of the blood volumes will provide correct information on the contents of the vascular bed. Measurements of the red cell mass are best performed with ^{99}Tc-labeled red cells (11). ^{125}I-labeled albumin is a useful plasma label for the plasma volume measurement (11).

The splenic red cell mass is measured using a quantitative scanning method (12, 13).

IRON STUDIES IN THE DIAGNOSIS OF MYELOFIBROSIS

Transferrin iron is taken up by red cell precursors and at the sites of iron storage (3). It is not taken up by the reticuloendothelial system (14). Thus, uptake of activity in the spleen during the hours following administration of radioactive iron indicates extramedullary erythropoiesis in the spleen. Iron uptake in the liver may be due either to uptake in the stores or to hepatic erythropoiesis (15, 16). Release of iron from the liver during the days following the injection of radioactive iron is suggestive of erythropoiesis in the liver. Occasionally, however, extramedullary erythropoiesis may be absent in myelofibrosis, although extramedullary leukopoiesis or thrombopoiesis is found (17). Furthermore, patients studied in the early stages of the disease may develop extramedullary erythropoiesis later during the course of the disease. Thus, failure to detect iron uptake in the spleen does not exclude PMF.

Diseases other than myelofibrosis which can also be associated with extramedullary erythropoiesis include chronic myeloid leukemia (18), chronic myelomonocytic leukemia (19), and widespread bone marrow involvement by carcinoma (20).

RESULTS OF ERYTHROKINETICS IN MYELOFIBROSIS

Red Cell Survival and Sites of Red Cell Destruction

The red cell survival of patients with PMF is usually shorter than normal. However, this shortening is not striking (17, 21, 22). A mean red cell life of less than 30 days was found in only 25% of the patients studied by Szur and Smith (17). The mean red cell life may even be normal (21). Najean and his colleagues showed that hemolysis was similar with autologous and isologous red cells (22), suggesting an extracorpuscular origin for the hemolysis. In some patients, immune hemolysis may contribute to the anemia (23).

Surface counting data (2, 17, 21, 24) suggest that in patients with PMF neither the spleen nor the liver plays a prominent role in red cell destruction.

Nevertheless, in the majority of the patients with PMF studied by Szur and Smith the spleen was more active as an organ of red cell destruction than was the liver (17). Nathan and Berlin (25) and Ward and Block (26) found definite uptake of red cells in the spleen. Christensen described increasing destruction of red cells in the spleen with increasing spleen size (27).

Ferrokinetics

Total Erythropoiesis

Ferrokinetic studies have shown that total erythropoietic activity is increased one to ten times in patients with PMF (17, 22, 28, 29). Erythroid failure may, however, occur in the terminal phase of the disease. Erythroid hypoplasia may also be associated with blastic transformation (30) and it can be a presenting feature (31). The overall incidence of erythroid hypoplasia in PMF is about 6%; it is associated with a bad prognosis (31).

Ineffective Erythropoiesis

Markedly increased iron turnover and a decreased red cell utilization of iron suggest that there is ineffective erythropoiesis in PMF (17, 22, 28, 29). In Najean's series, for instance, only 30% of the patients incorporated the injected radioiron normally (22).

^{59}Fe Surface-Counting Data

Surface counting is usually performed over the sacrum, the liver, and the spleen (Fig. 1). Normal iron uptake in the sacrum is rarely observed. In 30–80% of the patients no iron uptake in the sacrum could be detected (17, 22). By contrast, iron uptake in spleen and liver is found in at least 75% of the patients. Those in whom no iron uptake in the spleen can be detected are either in the earlier stages of the disease, or are suffering from myelofibrosis with red cell hypoplasia (31). The terminal phase of PMF, with burnt out erythropoiesis, may also be associated with absent radioiron uptake in the spleen.

Iron uptake is also found in the liver in two-thirds of the cases where it occurs in the spleen. On the other hand, erythropoiesis in the liver without erythropoiesis in the spleen is a rare event (28).

After administration of the ^{59}Fe, surface counts reach a plateau within a few hours. Thereafter, the radioactivity falls as ^{59}Fe labeled red cells leave the site of erythropoiesis. The rate of fall, which is dependent on the effectiveness of the erythropoiesis in the bone marrow, the spleen, or the liver, is usually of lesser magnitude than that observed from the sacrum curve in normal subjects (32). The rate of fall of the splenic radioactivity is influenced

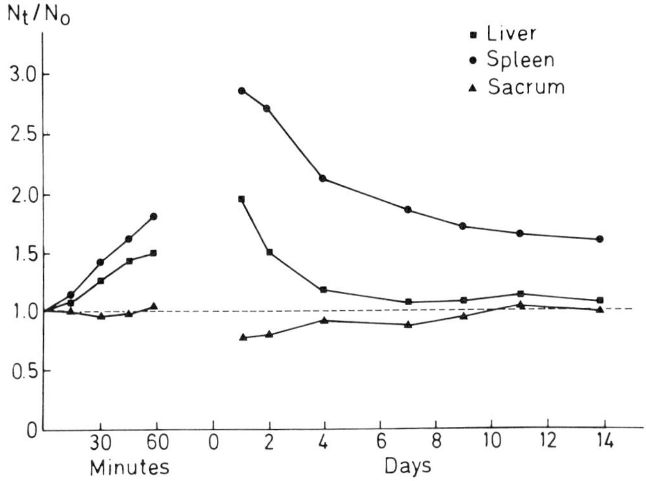

Figure 1 Surface-counting pattern following an intravenous injection of ^{59}Fe-transferrin into a patient with chronic primary myelofibrosis. There is little or no uptake by the bone marrow but a clear uptake by the spleen and the liver. The subsequent decrease in radioactivity over the liver is an indication that the iron is being used for erythropoiesis. Note that the decrease in radioactivity over the spleen is more delayed and incomplete as compared with the liver. This may be due to pooling or destruction of ^{59}Fe-labeled red cells in the spleen. Ineffective splenic erythropoiesis can also be responsible for incomplete release of ^{59}Fe from the spleen.

not only by the effectiveness of the splenic erythropoiesis, but also by pooling and/or destruction of newly labeled red cells in that organ.

As for the liver, iron that is taken up in the stores will be released much more slowly than iron taken up in hepatic red cell precursors; this causes uncertainties in interpreting the rate of hepatic iron release, especially when it is delayed.

To quantify more accurately the amount of ^{59}Fe that is effectively metabolized in the spleen, Christensen (33) has developed a method in which the observed surface counts are corrected for pooled radioactivity. This enables evaluation of the effective "clearing" of activity taken up by the spleen.

^{52}Fe Scanning

By contrast to the measurements at localized sites with ^{59}Fe, the use of ^{52}Fe makes it possible to visualize the sites of erythropoiesis over the whole body

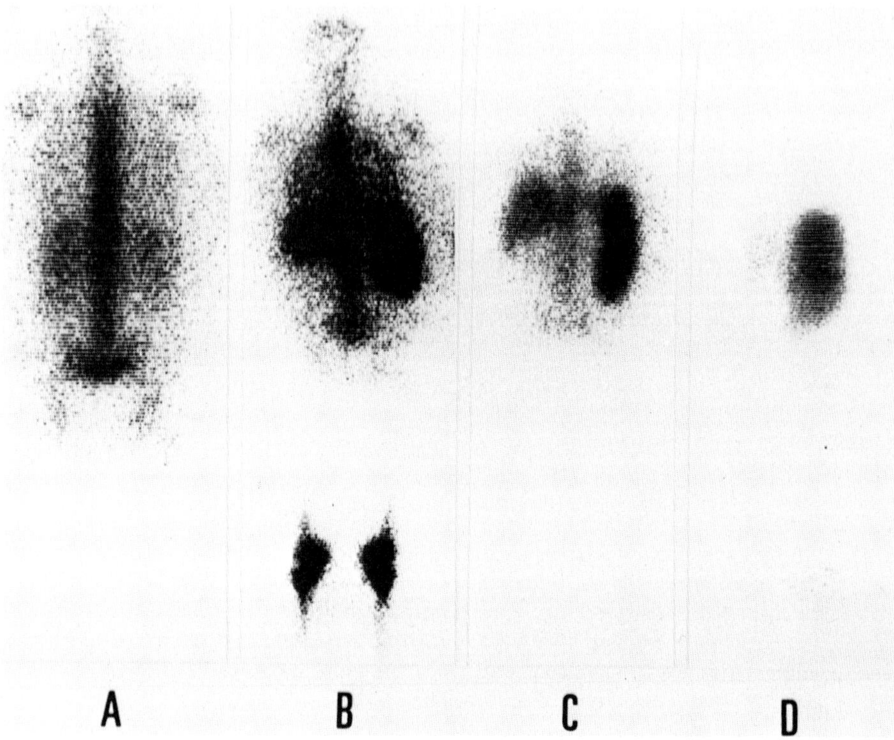

Figure 2 Examples of the distribution of active erythropoiesis in chronic primary myelofibrosis, as studied with ^{52}Fe. (A) Erythropoiesis in the usual areas with erythropoiesis in the spleen. (B) Marked erythropoiesis in the spleen with expansion of erythropoiesis in the long bones. (C) Lower than normal amount of erythropoiesis in the axial skeleton. Most of the radioiron is in the spleen and the liver. (D) Absence of erythropoiesis in the skeleton. Most of the injected iron is in the greatly enlarged spleen.

(Fig. 2). By this means, ^{52}Fe is capable of detecting extramedullary erythropoiesis. In a study of PMF, the ^{52}Fe scan did not show any uptake in the skeleton in a third of the patients (34). In these patients, almost all of the injected radioiron was taken up by the liver and the spleen. Iron uptake was sometimes observed in long bones, i.e., the humeri, femora, and tibiae, which are bone marrow expansion areas.

By quantitative scanning, the fraction of injected iron reaching the spleen, the liver, and the bone marrow can be measured (6, 34, 35). The fraction of iron taken up in the spleen ranged from 3 to 78% (6, 34), and the fraction of iron reaching the bone marrow ranged from 0 to 90% (34). The rate of iron uptake in the spleen, which should be closely related to the splenic erythropoiesis, ranged from 13 to 266 μmol/liter of blood/day (34). The higher value amounts to almost three times the normal marrow iron uptake rate.

Further interesting observations derived from ^{52}Fe scanning include suggestive evidence that bone marrow erythropoiesis is more effective than extramedullary erythropoiesis in PMF (35) and that in this disease the large erythropoietic spleen dominates iron uptake, thus restraining iron supply to the bone marrow (34). ^{52}Fe scanning also provided information that contributed to the description of the transitional myeloproliferative disorder syndrome (36).

ERYTHROKINETICS FOR PROGNOSIS IN MYELOFIBROSIS

PMF is a heterogeneous disorder, and the outcome of the disease varies greatly from case to case. Many workers have tried to relate findings at diagnosis with the clinical course. It is well established that anemia is an important factor in prognosis (37, 38). The hemoglobin value depends on both effective production of red cells and red cell destruction. It is also influenced by the expanded plasma volume and by the splenic red cell pool. Thus, additional information on these various factors in the pathogenesis of the anemia may be of interest for better defining the prognosis.

Najean and co-workers found that the degree of ineffective erythropoiesis, the amount of hemolysis, and the red cell mass were strongly related to the clinical course over the period of 1-2 years after the radionuclide investigations (22). In this study, ineffective erythropoiesis was defined as a red cell utilization below 60%, hemolysis as a rate of red cell destruction over 4%/day, and a low red cell mass as corresponding to a value below 80% of normal. Bentley and co-workers (28) and Barosi and co-workers (29) showed that erythroid failure was associated with a poor prognosis. Njoku and co-workers (35) have emphasized that the apparent anemia was largely dilutional, due to an enlarged plasma volume, and that this enlarged plasma volume (over 140% of predicted value) was a significant factor in prognosis. The amount of effective erythropoiesis is also of importance for prognosis. In this respect, Njoku and co-workers (35) have suggested that the bone marrow may contribute relatively more to effective erythropoiesis than do the spleen and the liver.

They found a positive correlation between medullary erythropoiesis and red cell mass.

To summarize, favorable prognostic factors include a near-normal red cell mass and plasma volume, no "excessive" hemolysis, satisfactory effective erythropoiesis without major ineffective erythropoiesis, and persistence of bone marrow erythropoiesis. All these favorable factors are more likely to be present early in the disease than later in its course.

SIGNIFICANCE OF ERYTHROKINETICS FOR TREATMENT

During the course of PMF, enlargement of the spleen almost always develops, often leading to functional or mechanical impairment. Splenomegaly influences the red cell count through hemodilution, an increased red cell pool and red cell destruction. For these reasons, it is often tempting to perform splenectomy or to treat by radiotherapy to the spleen. On the other hand, it has been believed that removal or irradiation of the spleen destroys an important area of blood formation and that the procedure could lead to harmful results (39). Even so, there is little doubt that splenectomy will increase the hemoglobin value provided there is adequate effective erythropoiesis in the bone marrow (and liver) (40). Thus, erythrokinetic studies should concentrate on measuring the effective erythropoiesis in bone marrow and liver if splenectomy is being considered for correction of the anemia. However, the evaluation of bone marrow erythropoiesis using ^{52}Fe in myelofibrosis may be misleading when an inadequate iron supply to the bone marrow is due to the spleen dominating iron uptake through intense erythropoiesis and a high blood flow (34). Accordingly, removal of the spleen will not only suppress a site of red cell pooling and red cell destruction, but it should also improve the iron supply to the bone marrow (41, 42).

Splenic irradiation for control of painful splenomegaly is useful in PMF (43). Moderate doses of radiotherapy delivered to the spleen have resulted in a marked improvement of the hematological status of two patients in whom ferrokinetics showed ineffective medullary and splenic erythropoiesis. The same treatment was ineffective or was even detrimental in seven other patients. None of the latter group had ineffective splenic and medullary erythropoiesis (44).

It has not yet been proved that splenectomy either increases survival or influences the course of the disease (45). Nevertheless, it is likely that the procedure could be of benefit to selected patients. In these, it might be reassuring to obtain ferrokinetic evidence of satisfactory effective erythropoiesis in bone marrow and liver before intervention, even if the rate of iron uptake in the bone marrow might lead to underestimation of the bone marrow erythropoiesis.

CONCLUSION

Erythrokinetic studies are helpful in PMF in many respects. Ferrokinetic studies may contribute to the diagnosis in demonstrating extramedullary erythropoiesis. Iron kinetics and red cell survival studies are of value in investigating the pathophysiology of the anemia which is a basic feature of this disease.

Prognosis may be better defined by these methods. Erythroid hypoplasia, largely ineffective erythropoiesis, intense hemolysis, and a large plasma volume are indicators of poor survival. Data from erythrokinetic studies might be of use for proposing a staging system.

Treatment of myelofibrosis may be influenced by the results of erythrokinetics. Persistence of satisfactory effective bone marrow erythropoiesis should be a reassuring feature when splenectomy is considered.

Finally, sequential evaluation of the erythropoiesis and its localization should provide a means for the comprehension of the development of extramedullary erythropoiesis in this disease.

REFERENCES

1. International Committee for standardization in haematology (ICSH). (1980). Recommended method for radioisotope red-cell survival studies. *Br. J. Haematol. 45*: 659–666.
2. Hughes-Jones, N. C., and Szur, L. (1957). Determination of the sites of red-cell destruction using ^{51}Cr-labelled cells. *Br. J. Haematol. 3*: 320–331.
3. Finch, C. A., Deubelbeiss, K., Cook, J. D., Eschbach, J. W., Harker, L. A., Funk, D. D., Marsaglia, G., Hillman, R. S., Slichter, S., Adamson, J. W., J. W., Ganzoni, A., and Giblett, E. R. (1970). Ferrokinetics in man. *Medicine 49*: 17–54.
4. Ricketts, C., Jacobs, A., and Cavill, J. (1975). Ferrokinetics and erythropoiesis in man. The measurement of effective erythropoiesis, ineffective erythropoiesis and red cell life span using ^{59}Fe. *Br. J. Haematol. 31*: 65–75.
5. François, P. E., and Szur, L. (1958). Use of Iron-52 as a radioactive tracer. *Nature 182*: 1665–1667.
6. Pettit, J. E., Lewis, S. M., Williams, E. D., Grafton, C. A., Bowring, C. S., and Glass, H. I. (1976). Quantitative studies of splenic erythropoiesis in polycythaemia vera and myelofibrosis. *Br. J. Haematol. 34*: 465–475.

7. Ferrant, A., Cauwe, F., Cogneau, M., Beckers, C., Verwilghen, R., and Sokal, G. (1980). Measurement of erythropoiesis using ^{52}Fe. *Br. J. Haematol. 45*: 447–457.
8. Chipping, P., Klonizakis, I., and Lewis, S. M. (1980). Indiumchloride scanning: a comparison with iron as a tracer for erythropoiesis. *Clin. Lab. Haematol. 2*: 255–263.
9. Motulski, A. G., Casserd, F., Giblett, E. R., Broun, G. O., and Finch, C. A. (1958). Anemia and the spleen. *New Engl. J. Med. 259*: 1164–1169.
10. McFadzean, A. J. S., Todd, D., and Tsang, K. C. (1958). Observations on the anemia of cryptogenetic splenomegaly. II. Expansion of the plasma volume. *Blood 13*: 524–532.
11. International Committee for standardization in haematology (ICSH). (1980). Recommended methods for measurement of red-cell and plasma volume. *J. Nucl. Med. 21*: 793–800.
12. Hegde, U. M., Williams, E. D., Lewis, S. M., Szur, L., Glass, H. I., and Pettit, J. E. (1973). Measurement of splenic red cell volume and visualisation of the spleen with ^{99m}Tc. *J. Nucl. Med. 14*: 769–771.
13. Ferrant, A., and Cauwe, F. (1979). Quantitative organ-uptake measurement with a gamma-camera. *Eur. J. Nucl. Med. 4*: 223–229.
14. Szur, L., Pettit, J. E., Lewis, S. M., Bruce-Tagoe, A. A., and Short, M. D. (1973). The effect of radiation on splenic function in myelosclerosis: studies with ^{52}Fe and ^{99}Tc^{m}. *Br. J. Radiol. 46*: 295–301.
15. Silverstein, M. N., Wolleager, E. E., and Baggenstoss, A. H. (1973). Gastrointestinal and abdominal manifestations of agnogenic myeloid metaplasia. *Arch. Intern. Med. 131*: 532–537.
16. Ligumski, M., Polliak, A., and Benbassat, J. (1978). Nature and incidence of liver involvement in agnogenic myeloid metaplasia. *Scand. J. Haematol. 21*: 81–93.
17. Szur, L., and Smith, M. D. (1961). Red-cell production and destruction in myelofibrosis. *Br. J. Haematol. 7*: 147–168.
18. Sjögren, V., and Brandt, L. (1974). Differences in morphology and mitotic activity between intra- and extra-medullary erythropoietic tissue in chronic myeloid leukaemia. *Scand. J. Haematol. 13*: 116–120.
19. Miescher, P. A., and Farquet, J. J. (1974). Chronic myelomonocytic leukemia in adults. *Semin. Hematol. 11*: 129–139.
20. Kiely, J. M., and Silverstein, M. N. (1969). Metastatic carcinoma simulating agnogenic myeloid metaplasia and myelofibrosis. *Cancer 24*: 1041–1044.
21. Pribilla, W., and Oettgen, H. F. (1968). Isotopenuntersuchungen bei Osteomyelofibrose. *Blut 18*: 178–182.
22. Najean, Y., Cacchione, R., Castro-Malaspina, H., and Dresh, C. (1978). Erythrokinetic studies in myelofibrosis: Their significance for prognosis. *Br. J. Haematol. 40*: 205–217.

23. Hasselbalch, H., Berild, D., and Hansen, O. P. (1984). Red-cell sensitization in myelofibrosis. *Scand. J. Haematol. 32*: 179–182.
24. Lewis, S. M., Szur, L., and Dacie, J. V. (1960). The pattern of erythrocyte destruction in haemolytic anaemias, as studied with radioactive chromium. *Br. J. Haematol. 6*: 122–139.
25. Nathan, D. G., and Berlin, N. I. (1959). Studies of the production and life span of erythrocytes in myeloid metaplasia. *Blood 14*: 668–682.
26. Ward, H. P., and Block, M. H. (1971). The natural history of agnogenic myeloid metaplasia (AMM) and a critical evaluation of its relationship with the myeloproliferative syndrome. *Medicine (Rochester) 50*: 357–420.
27. Christensen, B. E. (1975). Red cell kinetics. *Clin. Haematol. 4*: 393–405.
28. Szur, L., and Lewis, S. M. (1975). Iron kinetics. *Clin. Haematol. 4*: 407–425.
29. Barosi, G., Cazzola, M., Frassoni, F., Orlandi, E., and Stefanelli, M. (1981). Erythropoiesis in myelofibrosis with myeloid metaplasia: Recognition of different classes of patients by erythrokinetics. *Br. J. Haematol. 48*: 263–272.
30. Bentley, S. A., Murray, K. H., Lewis, S. M., and Roberts, P. D. (1977). Erythroid hypoplasia in myelofibrosis: A feature associated with blastic transformation. *Br. J. Haematol. 36*: 41–47.
31. Barosi, G., Baraldi, A., Cazzola, M., Spriano, P., and Magnini, U. (1983). Red cell aplasia in myelofibrosis with myeloid metaplasia. *Cancer (Philadelphia) 52*: 1290–1296.
32. Nakai, G. S., Craddock, C. G., and Figueroa, W. G. (1962). Agnogenic myeloid metaplasia. A survey of 29 cases and review of the literature. *Ann. Int. Med. 57*: 419–440.
33. Christensen, B. E. (1971). A new method for estimating splenic erythrocyte and plasma volume combined with quantitation of splenic iron incorporation. *Scand. J. Haematol. 8*: 245–249.
34. Ferrant, A., Rodhain, J., Cauwe, F., Cogneau, M., Beckers, C., Michaux, J. L., Verwilghen, R., and Sokal, G. (1982). Assessment of bone marrow and splenic erythropoiesis in myelofibrosis. *Scand. J. Haematol. 29*: 373–380.
35. Njoku, O. S., Lewis, S. M., Catovsky, D., and Gordon-Smith, E. C. (1983). Anaemia in myelofibrosis: Its value in prognosis. *Br. J. Haematol. 54*: 79–89.
36. Pettit, J. E., Lewis, S. M., and Nicholas, A. W. (1979). Transitional myeloproliferative disorder. *Br. J. Haematol. 43*: 167–184.
37. Silverstein, M. N. (1975). *Agnogenic myeloid metaplasia.* Acton, Publishing Sciences Group.
38. Meytes, D., Katz, D., and Ramot, B. (1976). Prognostic parameters in myeloid metaplasia: agnogenic versus postpolycythemia. *Israel J. Med. Sci. 12*: 534–542.

39. Doan, C. A. (1949). Hypersplenism. *Bull. N. Y. Acad. Med. 25*: 625–650.
40. Milner, G. R., Geary, C. G., Wadsworth, L. D., and Doss, A. (1973). Erythrokinetic studies as a guide to the value of splenectomy in primary myeloid metaplasia. *Br. J. Haematol. 25*: 467–484.
41. Wetherley-Mein, G., Jones, N. F., and Pullan, J. M. (1961). Effects of splenectomy on red cell production in myelofibrosis. *Br. Med. J. 1*: 84–89.
42. Tubiana, M., Parmentier, C., Lacour, J., and Mathé, G. (1966). Résultats d'explorations isotopiques pratiquées avant et après splénectomie. *Rev. Franç. Etudes Clin. et Biol. 11*: 790–805.
43. Greenberger, J. S., Chappey, J. T., Rosenthal, D. S., and Moloney, W. C. (1977). Irradiation for control of hypersplenism and painful splenomegaly in myeloid metaplasia. *Int. J. Rad. Oncol. Biol. Phys. 2*: 1083–1090.
44. Parmentier, C., Charbord, P., Tibi, M., and Tubiana, M. (1977). Splenic irradiation in myelofibrosis. Clinical findings and ferrokinetics. *Int. J. Rad. Oncol. Biol. Phys. 2*: 1075–1081.
45. Benbassat, J., Penchans, S., and Ligumski, M. (1979). Splenectomy in patients with agnogenic myeloid metaplasia: An analysis of 321 published cases. *Br. J. Haematol. 42*: 207–214.

7

Malignant or Acute Myelofibrosis

G. J. DEN OTTOLANDER
Leiden University Medical Center, Leiden, The Netherlands

INTRODUCTION

Myelofibrosis (or sclerosis) in general evokes the association of a chronic, prolonged process, which tends to obscure its fundamentally malignant character. The term "malignant myelosclerosis" was introduced in 1963 by Lewis and Szur (1) and located within the concept of the myeloproliferative disorders as described by Dameshek (2). The rapid clinical course and the physical and laboratory findings allowed a definite distinction of the picture from chronic (agnogenic) myelofibrosis. The variety of terms that have evolved from the literature to describe similar pictures or diseases that were supposed to be equivalent, e.g., acute myelofibrosis (3-15), acute myelosclerosis (16), malignant myelosclerosis (17-22), subacute myelosclerosis (23), and acute megakaryocytic myelofibrosis (24) obviously illustrate the confusion that developed about the precise definition of the disease and the controversy whether malignant or acute myelofibrosis exists as a clinicopathological entity.

In 1979 we published our findings in three patients with megakaryoblastic leukemia (25). From our own experience and reports describing similar pictures in the literature, we concluded that acute megakaryoblastic leukemia

(AMeL) appeared to be identical to acute myelofibrosis (AMF). In this chapter, the validity of the concept of AMF as a clinicopathological entity will be discussed, as will the diagnosis and differential diagnosis of the syndrome. Also, the recently altered therapeutic approaches will be surveyed.

ACUTE MYELOFIBROSIS: A CLINICOPATHOLOGICAL ENTITY?

Lewis and Szur (1) were the first authors to use the term "malignant myelosclerosis" to distinguish an acute rapidly progressive illness in five patients who showed the histological features of myelosclerosis from the terminal (acute) phase of chronic myelosclerosis. The syndrome was defined by rapidly developing pancytopenia, and the absence of enlargement of the liver, spleen, and lymph nodes. The blood smears showed only moderate abnormalities of the red blood cells and a few blasts in the white cell differential count. Bone marrow aspiration yielded a dry tap whereas the histological picture of a bone biopsy revealed increase in collagen tissue and argyrophil reticulin with a cellular picture that was dominated by round and oval mononuclear cells (probably primitive reticulum cells) and giant cells similar to megakaryocytes. The disease invariably ran a rapid downhill course. At necropsy, there were no signs of extramedullary hematopoiesis. The authors emphasized that this condition presents features of both myelosclerosis and leukemia, so that it must be distinguished from the acute terminal phase of chronic myelosclerosis and they discussed its relationship to the myeloproliferative disorders as proposed by Dameshek (2). Earlier, Wood and Andrews (23) published a report of three patients with "subacute myelosclerosis," but their data are insufficient to conclude that we are dealing with similar conditions.

After the introduction of the term "malignant myelosclerosis," several reports appeared describing the same or supposedly similar pictures, but they illustrate the confusion about the precise definition of the disease. A variety of synonyms have been used and a question arises concerning the validity of retaining malignant myelosclerosis as a disease entity.

Sanerkin (26), discussing the stromal changes in malignant bone marrow proliferations, stated that the occurrence of myelofibrosis does not signify an etiological relationship to the condition in which it occurs, and that there is no justification for the diagnosis of malignant myelofibrosis as a disease entity "solely upon the demonstration of increased reticulin fibrils and collagen fibrils" in cases which are, in fact, acute leukemia. Lubin et al. (22) believed that malignant myelosclerosis is best interpreted as an acute myeloproliferative disorder sharing features with acute leukemia and agnogenic myeloid metaplasia. Bird and Proctor (18) also "do not believe that there is enough evidence to separate malignant myelosclerosis from the pattern of acute leukemia." It was the opinion of Manoharan and Pitney (27) that malignant myelosclerosis may be but a variant of acute myeloblastic leukemia and that the distinction between AML with marrow fibrosis and malignant myelosclerosis is probably only of theoretical interest. Szur (28), however, again emphasized the uniqueness of malignant myelosclerosis in that it combines the blood and clinical picture akin to that of acute leukemia to a marrow picture of myelosclerosis with the characteristic proliferation of the megakaryopoiesis. The striking proliferation of atypical megakaryocytes was stressed by Fabich and Raich (7).

In 1979, Bearman et al. (29) published their data of seven patients with acute myelosclerosis, and carried out a thorough, critical review of the literature. In their opinion, only 13 of 49 patients published as such conformed to the criteria originally proposed for the disease. Once again these authors defined acute myelosclerosis as a distinct clinicopathological entity that can be separated from other myeloproliferative disorders. Their criteria were: pancytopenia with a few blast cells in the blood smear, absence of palpable lymph nodes and spleen, dry tap on bone marrow aspiration, a three-lineage proliferation in the bone marrow histology with predominance of the megakaryopoiesis, and no signs of extramedullary hematopoiesis. Although Lewis and Szur (1) did not emphasize the panmyelosis, the prominence of giant cells as described by them suggests the proliferation of the megakaryocytic cell line. A French publication (30) presented a selection from the literature that is almost identical to that included in the paper by Bearman et al. (29). In the same year, we (25) reported our findings in three patients with megakaryoblastic leukemia.

From our own experience and a study of the literature, we concluded that there were striking similarities between AMF and AMeL and we stated that the two pictures appeared to be identical. The criteria mentioned by Bearman et al. (29) were fully applicable to our patients. Cytological, cytochemical, and electron microscopical investigation of the blast cells of the peripheral blood strongly suggested their megakaryocytic origin. Convincing evidence that this hypothesis was valid has been provided by Breton-Gorius et al. (31) and Bain et al. (32) using the specific platelet peroxidase reaction. The common denominators of AMF and AMeL are: fibrosis of the marrow and proliferation of the megakaryocytic cell line. The former can be interpreted as a nonspecific secondary reaction to various stimuli and not as an integral part of the neoplastic process. Both cytogenetic (14) and glucose-6-phosphatase dehydrogenase studies (33) have shown the secondary character of the phenomenon, and the role of the megakaryocyte in the generation of fibrosis is discussed elsewhere in this volume (see p. 98). On the other hand, involvement of the megakaryocytic lineage is the specific phenomenon shared by AMF and AMeL. In the literature, the blast cells have not always been recognized as such and have been described under a variety of names, e.g., primitive reticulum cells, reticular blasts, and large primitive cells. Use of methylmethacrylate embedding for bone marrow histopathology (34) has enabled us to recognize these blast cells as immature cells of the megakaryopoietic line (see below).

In their paper, Bain et al. (32) support the view that AMeL is the most frequent underlying etiology of the clinical syndrome of AMF. Sultan et al. (35) proposed the name "acute myelodysplasia" with "myelofibrosis" for cases of pancytopenia without hepatosplenomegaly, and with a cellular bone marrow in which the three cell lines are dysmorphic with proliferation of blast cells and myelofibrosis without collagen formation. On the other hand, it has been suggested by other workers (36) that the term "megakaryoblastic leukemia" should be applied to cases with an almost exclusive proliferation of atypical and primitive megakaryocytes. We and others (1, 18, 25) have noted monolinear development as a terminal event, this possibly being the natural course of the disease. However the proliferation of three cell lines with predominance of the megakaryopoiesis is crucial for the diagnosis AMF. As fibrosis merely relates to a nonspecific reaction of the marrow and as AMF and AMeL are similar diseases, we prefer to designate this clinicopathological entity as acute megakaryoblastic leukemia. The relationship between acute myelodysplasia and myelofibrosis is further discussed in Chapter 8.

DIAGNOSIS AND COURSE

About 60 patients (including six patients from our own clinic) who fulfil the above-mentioned criteria have been reported in published papers under the two headings of AMF and AMeL. The disease can occur at any age, even in (very young) children (37-41). [The cases reported by Evans (6) do not fulfil the criteria in our opinion.] There seems to be a slight preponderance of males and the older age groups (Fig. 1), the median age for males (55 years) being slightly higher than for females (47.5 years). In the majority of the patients, there is a short history of unspecific complaints before the presentation with signs of anemia, bleeding disorders, or infection. Usually this period is no longer than 2-3 months. A story of long-existing hematological problems casts doubt on the diagnosis, although it does not rule it out. The physical findings are defined by the absence of overt organomegaly, but slight enlargement of the liver and/or the spleen is not incompatible with the diagnosis.

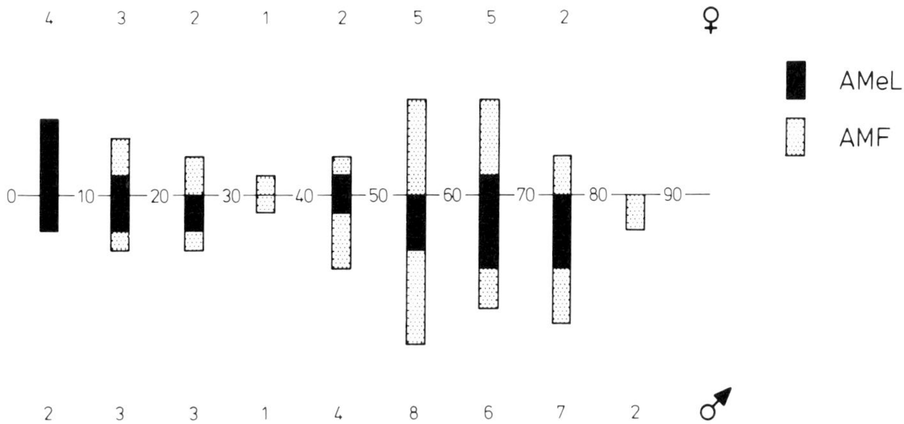

Figure 1 Age and sex distribution of acute myelofibrosis (AMF) and megakaryoblastic leukemia (AMeL). The data were obtained from published reports and the author's own cases (see text). Ages are indicated by the central row of figures; numbers of cases in each age group are given in the upper (for females) and lower (for males) rows.

The hematologic findings are those of pancytopenia (Table 1). Anemia below 10 g/dl was found in about 90% of the patients. The total white blood cell count was depressed (<4.0 × 10^9/liter) in 70% of cases and leukopenia below 1.0 × 10^9/liter was found in two-thirds of the patients, while one-third had values below 0.5 × 10^9/liter. Platelet counts above 100 × 10^9/liter were exceptional: this occurred in only 3 out of 59 patients; about 60% had platelet levels below 40 × 10^9/liter. The red blood cell picture shows only minor abnormalities; a few tear drop cells and erythroblasts are present. On the blood film, the white cell differential shows a decreased percentage of neutrophils, relative lymphocytosis, and some myeloid percursor cells. Blast cells can be noticed, but the percentage is usually low at diagnosis. Although the typical bleb-like extensions of the cytoplasm, together with the heavily packed, fine chromatin, may arouse suspicion that they are megakaryoblasts, their identification is not reliable with light microscopy alone (Fig. 2).

Cytochemistry, especially the periodic acid Schiff (PAS) and nonspecific esterase reactions (alpha naphthyl acetate esterase with diffuse multigranular pattern and negative alpha naphthyl butyrate esterase) can contribute to making the diagnosis. Recently, cytochemical demonstration of 5-nucleotidase activity has been reported as an important reaction to differentiate the megakaryoblast from blasts of other types of acute leukemia (42). However, convincing

Table 1 Hematological Findings in Acute Myelofibrosis (AMF) and Megakaryoblastic Leukemia (AMeL)

		Hemoglobin (g/dl)	TWBC ($\times 10^9$/liter)	Neutro ($\times 10^9$/liter)	Blasts (%)	Platelets ($\times 10^9$/liter)
Total population	Median	7.0	2.5	0.7	7	30
	Range	2.8–14	0.6–11.8	0–5.1	0–55	0–170
AMF	Median	6.6	2.2	0.5	8	30
	Range	2.8–14	0.6–11.8	0–2.0	0–55	0–170
AMeL	Median	7.2	3.1	0.8	2	30
	Range	3.6–12	0.6–8.6	0–5.1	0–49	0–130

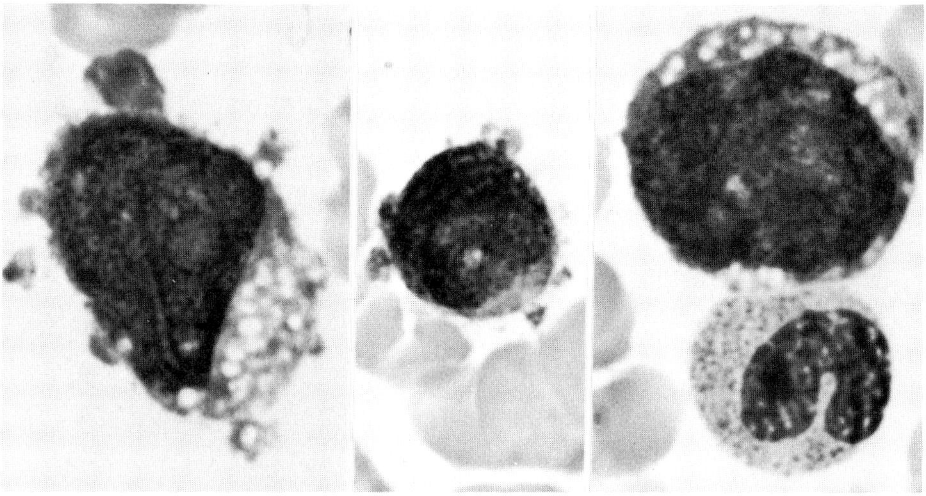

Figure 2 Blast cells (peripheral blood) that are strongly suspected to be of megakaryocytic origin.

evidence is obtained with the ultrastructural demonstration of the platelet peroxidase (PPO) (31). It is recommended that myeloperoxidase (MPO) reactions is carried out concomitantly, as myeloblasts also give a positive reaction with PPO, but the megakaryocytic cells are invariably negative with MPO (43). The use of platelet-specific monoclonal antibodies (anti-glycoproteins) has provided a promising method in distinguishing the blast cells (44–46). These markers become apparent on the very early cells of megakaryopoiesis, and remarkable correlation with the PPO reactions has been observed (47). Meticulous search of the peripheral blood for abnormal platelets results almost without exception in the detection of dysplastic platelets as described by Maldonado et al. (48) in the myeloproliferative syndrome. These abnormalities have been reported by us (49), and very recently platelet dysfunction in AMeL has been documented by others (38, 50). Additional evidence of megakaryoblastic proliferation is the finding of an increased serum lactodehydrogenase level with an isomorphic isoenzyme pattern (25, 38).

Marrow aspiration usually results in a dry tap. However, investigation of the small amount of material which is obtained may reveal dysplastic megakaryocytes and blast cells. Pancytopenia with dry tap on marrow aspiration makes biopsy histology essential. By this procedure, the marrow shows a hypercellular picture dominated by atypical megakaryocytes and large blast-

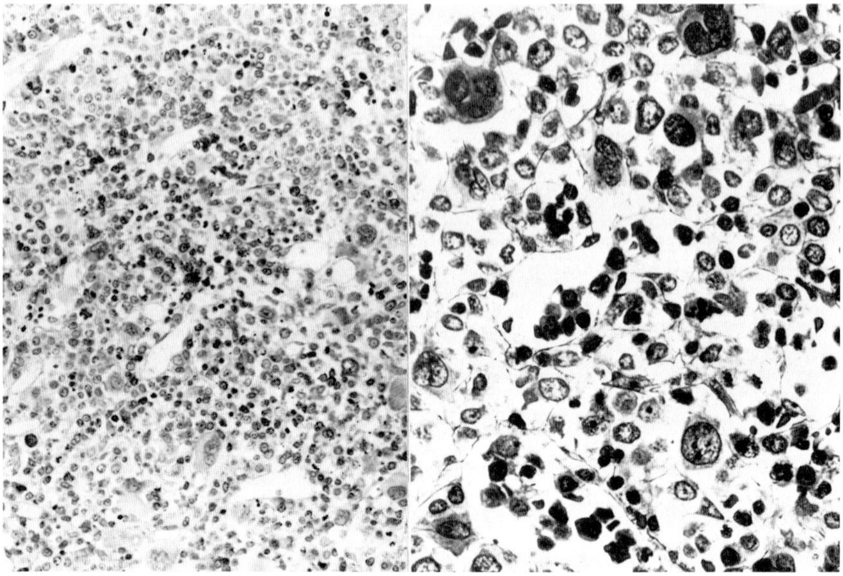

Figure 3 Bone marrow biopsy: hypercellular marrow with predominance of atypical megakaryocytes, blast cells, and slight reticulin fibrosis. Methyl-methacrylate, Gallamine Giemsa, and Gomori's reticulin stains, 200 and 400X. (Courtesy of Dr. J. te Velde.)

like cells (Fig. 3). With the methyl-methacrylate technique, recognition of the blast cells as the product of megakaryopoiesis has become possible. Especially noteworthy is the presence of block-like PAS-positivity located at the periphery of the cytoplasm, as this presents a typical picture. Proliferation of immature members of the granulocytic series and dysmorphic erythropoiesis are also observed.

The three-lineage hyperplasia is a special feature of AMF. In two of our patients, we noticed a large amount of lymphoid inflammatory infiltrate during the early phase of the disease. Increase of reticulin fibrils may be limited in the very beginning, and this allows aspiration of (scanty) marrow particles. Fiber content increases during the course of the disease (Fig. 3) and collagen formation becomes evident, but osteomyelosclerosis with extensions of bone trabecules and myeloid metaplasia argue against the diagnosis.

A diversity of cytogenetic abnormalities have been described in AMF and AMeL, but in the majority of these the patients did not fulfil the diagnostic criteria, or insufficient information was given to confirm the diagnosis (14,

20, 51-54). In our patients, we observed trisomy of chromosome 10 in one, a 47XY+? and 48XY+?+? in another, a translocation t1,3 in a third, and tetra- and octaploid metaphases in the fourth. Further abnormal patterns reported are: a marker chromosome one (9, 40), trisomy of chromosomes 2, 8, 12, 19, and 21 (singular or various combinations), and translocation of the long arm of the 21st to the 11th chromosome (40). The last report discusses the relationship of abnormalities of chromosome 21 to AMeL and supposes that trisomy 21 may predispose not only to ALL and ANLL but also to other hematopoietic disorders; this suggestion was also made by Lewis et al. (41) who reported a 3-year old boy with AMeL, trisomy 21, and marker chromosome (?Bq+). A ring 21 chromosome has been described in a 31-month-old boy with AMeL (38).

Although improved supportive care may have added to a longer course, the disease runs a rapidly downhill course in the vast majority of the patients. Until a few years ago (see below), the median survival was about 5 months (range, <1-22 months). Usually pancytopenia persists, with increasing blast cell counts. Development of a frankly leukemic blood picture with high leukocyte counts has been noticed (1, 18, 25, 29). The blast cell population may be of mixed composition (myelo-, erythro-, and megakaryoblasts). As in acute leukemia, infections and bleeding disorders are the most frequent causes of death. The findings at autopsy vary according to the development of the disease. The bone marrow histology can reveal the original picture unchanged or may show progressively increased fiber content, or, in case of leukemic development, a dense infiltrate of blast cells each surrounded by a fine meshwork of reticulin fibrils. Leukemic infiltration may be observed in almost every organ, including lymph nodes. However, myeloid metaplasia is not part of the picture. Remarkably, in one of our patients and in patient 5 of Bearman, the spleen was infiltrated diffusely by (chloroacetate esterase positive) myeloblasts.

Secondary development of AMF has been described after idiopathic acquired sideroblastic anemia (15, 55) or cytostatic therapy (11, 56, 57). However, the patients in these reports do not satisfy the diagnostic criteria. Furthermore, we have noticed the development of AMeL in patients with Hodgkin's disease after chemo- and radiotherapy (unpublished).

Differential Diagnosis (See Table 2)

The clinical picture of AMF/AMeL has an extensive differential diagnosis. From the pathologist's point of view, the observation of fibrosis in the marrow is crucial and leaves a limited number of possibilities. It is essential to know whether there is a hypercellular or a hypocellular picture. If the

Table 2 Differential Diagnosis of Acute Myelofibrosis

	AMF	PMF	CML	AL	HCL	FNM	AA	CAR
Clinical course	Acute	Chronic	Chronic	Acute	Chronic	Acute or Chronic	Acute or Chronic	Undefinable
Peripheral blood								
pancytopenia	++	–	–	–/±	+/++	+/++	++	–/±
blast cells	+	±	±	+/++	–	±	–	±
RBC abnormal	–	+/++	±	±	+	–	+	+/++
Bone marrow								
dry tap	++	+/++	±	±	+/++	+	±	±
cellularity	++	±/++	++	++	+/++	–	–	+
megakaryocytes	++	+/++	+/++	–	–/+	–	–	+/++
fibrosis	++	++/+++*	+	±	++	+	–	+
Physical findings								
hepatosplenomegaly	–	++	+	±	++	–	–	±

– = Absent/decreased; ± = possible/slightly decreased; + = present/normal; ++ = evident/increased; * = osteomyelosclerosis. See text for explanation of abbreviations.

marrow is hypercellular, all types of leukemia and myeloproliferative diseases must be taken into account. When there is a hypocellular marrow, one should consider autoimmune myelitis; in this the fibrosis shows a typical perivascular distribution and a picture recently described by our group as fibrosing necrotizing myelitis (FNM) (58). This entity is defined by a hypocellular marrow with an inflammatory infiltrate, vascular necrosis, interstitial fibrosis, and foci of residual hematopoiesis with scarcity of megakaryopoiesis. A considerable percentage (about 80%) of these patients, who present with pancytopenia, develop overt acute nonlymphatic leukemia. A minority remain pancytopenic. It should be stressed that this picture fits confusingly well in the concept of AMF.

The clinician may find it difficult to discriminate AMF from the following conditions:

1. *Primary Chronic Myelofibrosis (PMF),* especially the terminal events whether leukemic or cytopenic. A thorough history will disclose a long period of complaints in most patients. Splenomegaly is almost always present. Pancytopenia is an exception but may develop ultimately. The leukoerythroblastic picture of the peripheral blood with the striking red cell abnormalities of teardrop poikilocytes point to the correct diagnosis. Although the bone marrow biopsy pictures for PMF and AMF may appear indistinguishable (trilinear proliferation and fibrosis), the appearance in the latter is more immature, and osteomyelosclerosis with bone extensions are strong arguments against the diagnosis AMF.

2. *Chronic myeloid leukemia (CML)* with marrow fibrosis should not offer serious problems in the differential diagnosis. The peripheral blood picture with the complete maturation line of the leukocytes, the basophilia, and the detection of the Philadelphia chromosome in the majority of CML patients together with splenomegaly are indicative. Sometimes, in the course of CML, myelofibrosis increases and the picture may become indistinguishable from PMF (59, 60). The blast crisis of CML can present with dry tap and myelofibrosis, and in case of megakaryoblastic type (61) it may cause problems in differentiating it from AMeL.

3. *Acute leukemia (AL) with fibrosis.* This subject has been discussed extensively in the first part of this chapter. Marrow fibrosis can be observed in diverse acute leukemias, myeloid as well as nonmyeloid, and several authors have commented on this problem (26, 62, 63). The overt leukemic development in some cases of AMF especially may cause serious problems. Weisenburger (37) states that a biopsy specimen should be taken early in the course of the disease because at a later stage the picture may become indistinguishable from acute leukemia with fibrosis, when the disorder evolves toward overt leukemia.

4. *Hairy cell leukemia (HCL) and aplastic anemia (AA)* theoretically will be included in the differential diagnosis. If the typical hairy cell cannot be detected by scrutiny of the peripheral blood, the bone marrow biopsy will reveal a picture that differs essentially from that seen in AMF. Actually, AA should not pose any problem in differential diagnosis as fibrosis is incompatible with the diagnosis of AA, and the bone marrow biopsy will show an empty marrow. However, in some aplastic patients [grade II of Te Velde (64)], the marrow is atypical with marked fibrosis, and in this group several patients have developed frank leukemia (65).

Recently we have investigated a patient (62-year-old male) whose history illustrates the difficulties that may arise in diagnosis.

> The patient was referred with the diagnosis aplastic anemia. There was a 2-week history of increasing tiredness and hemorrhagic diathesis. Physical examination revealed no organomegaly. The peripheral blood showed severe pancytopenia (Hb 7 g/dl, WBC 0.9×10^9/liter, platelets 5×10^9/liter), there were slight abnormalities of the red blood cells (poikilocytes) and an occasional large vacuolated blast cell was observed. The scarce material obtained by marrow aspiration revealed dysmorphic members of three cell lines, and dispersed through the material were very large blast cells, the majority of which were heavily vacuolated, some reminiscent of megakaryocytic differentiation. The picture was interpreted as being definitely malignant, and a diagnosis of AMeL or AMF was suggested. The bone marrow biopsy, surprisingly, showed the picture of a fibrosing necrotizing myelitis, with an excess of blast cells of three cell lines and scarity of megakaryocytes.

5. *Bone marrow infiltration of diverse carcinomas* (CAR) can mimic the clinical picture of AMF. Myelofibrosis due to carcinoma metastases has been reported in the literature (66, 67). The presence of leukoerythroblastosis in the peripheral blood will help in differentiating these cases from AMF.

THERAPY

Until a few years ago, in general therapy was limited to the application of mild chemotherapy and supportive care. Various drugs have been used (azathioprine, busulphan, cyclophosphamide, cytosine arabinoside, 6-mercaptopurin, prednisone, 6-thioguanine, and vincristine), separately or in various combinations, each with disappointing outcome. Survival has been severely limited and complete remissions were not obtained. Recently a, more aggressive policy has been adopted; this has resulted in several complete remissions, and the prognosis of this usually rapidly fatal disease has improved substantially. The two major goals have been (a) the use of anthracyclin derivatives and (b) bone marrow transplantation. In 1981 Bain et al. (32) reported the achievement of a complete remission and a 5^+ months survival with a combination of daunorubicin, cytosine arabinoside, and 6-thioguanine (DAT protocol) in a 14-year-old girl with AMeL. Several publications followed, confirming the efficacy of the anthracyclins (38-40, 68, 69). In our series of six patients, we obtained a partial remission with daunorubicin and a total survival of 22 months (compared with a median of 5 months, range 3-7 months, in the others who were treated with limited chemotherapy). Although no definitive conclusions can be drawn from these limited studies, the results with the anthracyclins appear to be very promising with a median survival of 12^+ months (range 5^+-22 months) obtained in eight patients. Bone marrow transplantation has been advocated for AMF and AMeL (68, 70-72). The limited number of patients allows only speculation about the impact of this treatment on the prognosis, but four (out of seven) patients have remitted after bone marrow transplantation, with a median survival to date of 10 months (range 5^+-15^+ months). Both forms of therapy have one remarkable phenomenon in common; namely, the disappearance of fibrosis after treatment (39, 68, 70, 71). This had been noticed previously (37) with another therapeutic schedule, and reversal of fibril content after chemotherapy has been mentioned by others (62) in acute lymphatic and nonlymphatic leukemias.

CONCLUSION

The designation "malignant myelosclerosis" has been applied to a heterogenous group of hematological malignancies. The extensive use of synonyms has led to much confusion. The validity of retaining the syndrome as a well-defined clinicopathological entity has been questioned and other synonyms were proposed. In our opinion, continued use of these eponyms complicates the situation. As "malignant myelosclerosis" emphasizes an unspecific fibrotic reaction, we prefer the name "acute megakaryoblastic leukemia," which focuses on the crucial requisite of this panmyelotic myeloproliferative disorder, i.e., predominance of the dysmorphic megakaryopoiesis. New diagnostic tools (plastic embedding of bone biopsies, platelet peroxidase reaction, anti-platelet monoclonal antibodies) have improved identification of the blast cells and have provided an important contribution to the differential diagnosis of this pancytopenic disorder. The remarkable successes obtained with the anthracyclins make these cytostatics the therapeutic agents of choice. Results with bone marrow transplantation are yet preliminary and further experiences should be awaited in order to assess the advantages, if any, of this treatment.

REFERENCES

1. Lewis, S. M., and Szur, L. (1963). Malignant myelosclerosis. *Br. Med. J. 2*: 472–477.
2. Dameshek, W. (1951). The myeloproliferative syndromes. *Blood 6*: 372–375.
3. Bergsman, K. L., and Van Slyck, E. J. (1971). Acute myelofibrosis. An accelerated variant of agnogenic myeloid metaplasia. *Ann. Intern. Med. 74*: 232–235.
4. Breton-Gorius, J., Daniel, M. T., Flandrin, G., and Denoel, G. K. (1973). Fine structure and peroxidase activity of circulating micromegakaryoblasts and platelets in a case of acute myelofibrosis. *Br. J. Haematol. 25*: 331–339.
5. Brière, J., Castro-Malaspina, H., Brière, J. F., and Bernard, J. (1976). Les myelofibroses aiguës ou subaiguës. *Nouv. Rev. Fr. Hematol. 16*: 3–22.
6. Evans, D. I. K. (1975). Acute myelofibrosis in children with Down's syndrome. *Arch. Dis. Child. 50*: 458–462.
7. Fabich, D. R., and Raich, P. C. (1977). Acute myelofibrosis. A report of three cases. *Am. J. Clin. Pathol. 67*: 334–338.
8. Libnoch, J. A., Ajlouni, K., Millman, W. L., Guansing, A. R., and Theil, G. B. (1977). Acute myelofibrosis and malignant hypercalcemia. *Am. J. Med. 62*: 432–438.
9. Mitus, W. J., Coleman, N., and Kiossoglou, K. A. (1969). Abnormal (marker) chromosomes in two patients with acute myelofibrosis. *Arch. Intern. Med. 123*: 192–197.
10. Patel, A. R., Shah, P. C., and Rhee, H. L. (1976). Acute myelofibrosis and acute myeloblastic leukaemia. *Br. Med. J. 2*: 1232.
11. Pinedo, H. M., van Hemel, J. O., Vrede, M. A., and van der Sluys Veer, J. (1974). Acute myelofibrosis and chromosome damage after procarbazine treatment. *Br. Med. J. 3*: 525.
12. Spector, J. I., and Levine, P. H. (1973). Case report. Carcinomatous bone marrow invasion simulating acute myelofibrosis. *Am. J. Med. Sci. 266*: 145–148.
13. Takacsi-Nagy, L., and Graf, F. (1975). Definition, clinical features and diagnosis of myelofibrosis. *Clin. Haematol. 4*: 291–308.
14. Van Slyck, E. J., Weiss, L., and Dully, M. (1970). Chromosomal evidence for the secondary role of fibroblastic proliferation in acute myelofibrosis. *Blood 36*: 729–735.
15. Yeung, K. Y., and Trowbridge, A. A. (1977). Idiopathic acquired sideroblastic anemia terminating in acute myelofibrosis. Case report and review of literature. *Cancer 39*: 359–365.
16. Dameshek, W., and Gunz, F. (1958). Leukemia and the "myeloproliferative" disorders. In *Leukemia*. New York, Grune & Stratton, pp. 262–297.

17. Aufdermauer, M. (1964). Osteomyelosklerose: Chronische und maligne Verlaufsform. *Fortschr. Geb. Roentgenstr. Nuklearmed 101*: 66–68.
18. Bird, T., and Proctor, S. J. (1977). Malignant myelosclerosis. Myeloproliferative disorder or leukemia? *Am. J. Clin. Pathol. 67*: 512–520.
19. Castleman, B., and McNeely, B. U., eds. (1966). Case records of the Massachusetts General Hospital. *N. Engl. J. Med. 274*: 1200–1208.
20. Khan, M. H., and Martin, H. (1968). Multiple chromosomal aberrations in a case of malignant myelosclerosis. *Acta Haematol. 39*: 299–308.
21. Lewis, S. M., and Szur, L. (1974). Blood and neoplastic diseases. Myeloproliferative disorders. *Br. Med. J. 4*: 399–402.
22. Lubin, J., Rozen, S., and Rywlin, A. M. (1976). Malignant myelosclerosis. *Arch. Intern. Med. 136*: 141–145.
23. Wood, E. E., and Andrews, C. T. (1949). Subacute myelosclerosis. Report of three cases. *Lancet ii*: 739–743.
24. Estevez, J. M., Urueta, E. E., and Moran, T. J. (1974). Acute megakaryocytic myelofibrosis. Case report of an unusual myeloproliferative syndrome. *Am. J. Clin. Pathol. 62*: 52–59.
25. Den Ottolander, G. J., Te Velde, J., Brederoo, P., Geraedts, J. P. M., Slee, P. H. T., Willemze, R., Zwaan, F. E., Haak, H. L., Muller, H. P., and Bieger, R. (1979). Megakaryoblastic leukaemia (acute myelofibrosis): A report of three cases. *Brit. J. Haematol. 42*: 9–20.
26. Sanerkin, N. G. (1964). Stromal changes in leukaemic and related bone marrow proliferations. *J. Clin. Pathol. 17*: 541–547.
27. Manoharan, A., Pitney, W. R. (1977). Acute myeloblastic leukaemia with marrow fibrosis (malignant myelosclerosis): Acute leukaemia or malignant myelosclerosis? *Aust. N.Z.J. Med. 7*: 638–641.
28. Szur, L. (1974). In Dahlem Workshop on myelofibrosis-osteosclerosis syndrome. Berlin 1974. *Advances in the Biosciences*, vol. 16. Edited by R. Burkhardt et al., Vieweg, Pergamon Press, p. 251.
29. Bearman, R. M., Pangalis, G. A., and Rappaport, H. (1979). Acute ("malignant") myelosclerosis. *Cancer 43*: 279–293.
30. Lefèvre, P., Ricard, H. F., Imbert, M., Reyes, F., Pinalideau, Y., and Sultan, C. (1979). La myelofibrose maligne. Une observation. *Nouv. Presse Med. 8*: 3545–3547.
31. Breton-Gorius, J., Reyes, F., Duhamel, G., Najman, A., and Gorin, N. C. (1978). Megakaryoblastic leukemia: identification by ultrastructural demonstration of platelet peroxidase. *Blood 51*: 45–60.
32. Bain, B. J., Catovsky, D., O'Brien, M., Grant Prentice, H., Lawlor, E., Kumaran, T. O., McCann, S. R., Matutes, E., and Galton, D. A. G. (1981). Megakaryoblastic leukemia presenting as acute myelofibrosis—A study of four cases with the platelet peroxidase reaction. *Blood 58*: 206–213.
33. Greenberg, B. R., Wilson, F. D., Woo, L., and Jenks, H. M. (1978). Cytogenetics of fibroblastic colonies in Ph^1-positive chronic myelogenous leukemia. *Blood 51*: 1039–1044.

34. Te Velde, J., Burkhardt, R., Kleiverda, K., Leenheers-Binnendijk, L., and Sommerfeld, W. (1977). Methyl-methacrylate embedding medium in histopathology. *Histopathology 1*: 319–330.
35. Sultan, C., Sigaux, F., Imbert, M., and Reyes, F. (1981). Acute myelodysplasia with myelofibrosis: A report of eight cases. *Br. J. Haematol. 49*: 11–16.
36. Mirchandani, I., and Palutke, M. (1983). Acute megakaryoblastic leukemia. *Cancer 50*: 2866–2872.
37. Weisenburger, D. D. (1980). Acute myelofibrosis terminating as acute myeloblastic leukemia. *Am. J. Clin. Pathol. 73*: 128–132.
38. Pui, C. H., Williams, D. L., Scarborough, V., Jackson, C. W., Price, R., and Murphy, S. (1982). Acute megakaryoblastic leukaemia associated with intrinsic plateled dysfunction and constitutional ring 21 chromosome in a young boy. *Br. J. Haematol. 50*: 191–200.
39. Breton-Gorius, J., Bizet, M., Reyes, F., Du Puy, E., Mear, C., Vannier, J. P., and Tron, P. (1982). Myelofibrosis and acute megakaryoblastic leukemia in a child: Topographic relationship between fibroblasts and megakaryocytes with an α-granule effect. *Leuk. Res 6*: 97–110.
40. Chan, W. C., Brynes, R. K., Kim, T. H., Verras, A., Schick, C., Green, R. J., and Ragad, A. H. (1983). Acute megakaryoblastic leukemia in early childhood. *Blood 62*: 92–98.
41. Lewis, D. S., Thompson, M., Hudson, E., Liberman, M. M., and Samson, D. (1983). Down's syndrome and acute megakaryoblastic leukaemia. *Acta Haematol. 70*: 236–242.
42. El-Mohandes, E., and Hayhoe, F. G. J. (1983). 5-Nucleotidase activity of megakaryoblasts in a case of acute megakaryoblastic leukaemia. *Br. J. Haematol. 53*: 523–526.
43. Parkin, J. L., Mc Kenna, R. W., and Brunning, R. D. (1982). Philadelphia chromosome-positive blastic leukaemia:ultrastructural and ultracytochemical evidence of basophil and mast cell differentiation. *Br. J. Haematol. 52*: 663–667.
44. McMichael, A. J., Rust, N. A., Pilch, J. R., Solchynsky, R., Morton, J., Mason, D. Y., Ruan, C., Tobelem, G., and Caen, J. (1981). Monoclonal antibody to human platelet glycoprotein I. I. Immunological studies. *Br. J. Haematol. 49*: 501–509.
45. Vainchenker, W., Deschamps, J. F., Bastin, J. M., Guichard, J., Titeux, M., Breton-Gorius, J., and McMichael, A. J. (1982). Two monoclonal anti-platelet antibodies as markers of human megakaryocyte maturation. Immunofluorescent staining and platelet peroxidase detection in megakaryocyte colonies and in vivo cells from normal and leukemic patients. *Blood 59*: 514–521.
46. Bevan, D., Rose, M., and Greaves, M. (1982). Leukaemia of platelet precursors: diverse features in four cases. *Br. J. Haematol. 51*: 147–164.

47. Breton-Gorius, J., Fabillio, A., Vainchenker, W., Vinci, G., Van Haeke, D., Henri, A., Guichard, J., and Canizo, M. C. (1983). Diagnosis of megakaryoblastic leukemias. *Verh. Dtsch. Ges. Path. 67*: 166–181.
48. Maldonado, J. E., Pintado, T., and Pierre, R. V. (1974). Dysplastic and circulating megakaryocytes in chronic myeloproliferative disease: I The platelets: Ultrastructural and peroxidase reaction. *Blood 43*: 797–809.
49. Den Ottolander, G. J., Brederoo, P., and Te Velde, J. (1979). Megakaryoblastic leukaemia: Morphology of megakaryoblasts and platelets. *Abstract Proc. Int. Soc. Haematol., Europ. & Afric. division, Fifth meeting I*: 31.
50. Hendrick, A. M., Shah, S., and Raich, P. C. (1984). Platelet dysfunction in acute megakaryoblastic leukemia. *Arch. Pathol. Lab. Med. 108*: 63–64.
51. Nowell, P., Jensen, J., Gardner, F., Murphy, S., Changanti, R. S. K., and German, J. (1976). Chromosome studies in "preleukemia." III. Myelofibrosis. *Cancer 38*: 1873–1881.
52. Bartoli, E., Massarelli, G., Soggia. G., Tanda, F., and Vianello, M. G. (1979). Acute agnogenic myeloid metaplasia with chromosomal abnormalities. *Acta Haematol. 62*: 206–213.
53. Shah, I., Mayeda, K., Koppitch, F., Mahmood, S., and Nemitz, B. (1982). Karyotypic polymorphism in acute myelofibrosis. *Blood 60*: 841–844.
54. Berrebi, A., Dvilanski, A., and Chemke, J. (1982). Cytogenetic studies in megakaryoblastic leukaemia. *Acta Haematol. 69*: 66–67.
55. Butler, W. M., Taylor, H. G., and Viswanathan, U. (1982). Idiopathic acquired sideroblastic anemia terminating in acute myelosclerosis. *Cancer 49*: 2497–2499.
56. Gisser, S. D., and Chung, K. B. (1979). Acute myelofibrosis in progressive systemic sclerosis. Report of a case developing during long-term chlorambucil therapy and discussion of pathogenetic factors. *Am. J. Med. 67*: 151–154.
57. Ali, N. O., and Janes, W. O. (1979). Malignant myelosclerosis (acute myelofibrosis): Report of two cases following cytotoxic chemotherapy. *Cancer 43*: 1211–1215.
58. Te Velde, J., and Spaander, P. J. (1982). Aplastic anaemia and myelodysplastic syndrome: Differential diagnosis. *Presented at the 19th Congress of the Int. Soc. Haemat. Budapest.*
59. Buyssens, N., and Bourgeois, N. H. (1977). Chronic myelocytic leukemia versus idiopathic myelofibrosis: A diagnostic problem in bone marrow biopsies. *Cancer 40*: 1548–1561.
60. Clough, V., Geary, C. G., Hashmi, K., Davson, J., and Knowlson, T. (1979). Myelofibrosis in chronic granulocytic leukaemia. *Br. J. Haematol. 42*: 515–526.
61. Bain, B., Catovsky, D., O'Brien, M., Spiers, A. S. D., and Richards,

H. G. H. (1979). Megakaryoblastic transformation of chronic granulocytic leukaemia. An electron microscopy and cytochemical study. *J. Clin. Pathol. 30*: 235–242.
62. Manoharan, A., Horsley, R., and Pitney, W. R. (1979). The reticulin content of bone marrow in acute leukaemia in adults. *Br. J. Haematol. 43*: 185–190.
63. Ghandour, C., LePrisé, P. Y., and Ramée, M. P. (1981). La myélofibrose au cours des leucémies aiguës. *Nouv. Rev. Fr. Hematol. 23*: 219–225.
64. Te Velde, J., and Haak, H. L. (1978). Aplastic anaemia in adults. Histological investigation of methacrylate embedded biopsy specimens; correlation with survival after conventional treatment in 15 adult patients. *Br. J. Haematol. 35*: 61–69.
65. Te Velde, J., and Haak, H. L. (1979). Histology in bone marrow failure, a follow-up study in aplastic anaemia. *Haematol. Bloodtransfusion 24*: 15–24.
66. Spector, J. I., and Levine, P. H. (1973). Carcinomatous bone marrow invasion simulating acute myelofibrosis. *Am. J. Med. Sci. 266*: 145–148.
67. Kiang, D., Mc Kenna, R., and Kennedy, B. (1978). Reversal of myelofibrosis in advanced breast cancer. *Am. J. Med. 64*: 173–176.
68. Metha, A. B., Baughan, A. S. J., Catovsky, D., Goldman, J. M., Johnson, S. A., and Galton, D. A. G. (1983). Reversal of marrow fibrosis in acute megakaryoblastic leukaemia after remission-induction and consolidation chemotherapy followed by bone marrow transplantation. *Br. J. Haematol. 53*: 445–449.
69. Strebel, U., Schabner, A., and Fehr, J. (1983). Die akute Osteomyelofibrose. *Schweiz. med. Wschr. 113*: 844–850.
70. Smith, J. W., Shulman, H. M., Thomas, E. D., Fefer, A., and Buckner, C. D. (1981). Bone marrow transplantation for acute myelosclerosis. *Cancer 48*: 2198–2203.
71. Wolf, J. L., Spruce, W. E., Bearman, R. M., Forman, S. J., Scott, E. P., Fahey, J. L., Farbstein, M. J., Rappaport, H., and Blume, K. G. (1982). Reversal of acute ("malignant") myelosclerosis by allogeneic bone marrow transplantation. *Blood 59*: 191–193.
72. Rozman, C., Grañena, A., Hernàndez-Prieto, M., Vela, E., and Brugués, R. (1982). Bone marrow transplantation for acute myelofibrosis. *Lancet i*: 618.

8

Acute Myelodysplasia With Myelofibrosis

F. SIGAUX, M. IMBERT, AND C. SULTAN
Service Central d'Hématologie-Immunologie, Hôpital Henri Mondor, Creteil, France

INTRODUCTION

As described in Chapter 7, in 1963, Lewis and Szur (1) published five cases termed "malignant myelosclerosis." Since then many papers have been published referring to that initial description (see p. 140). Unfortunately, the subject has been difficult to elucidate because of various problems, inter alia (a) a problem of terminology, as different authors successively changed the initial designation of "malignant myelosclerosis," eventually arriving at the term "acute myelofibrosis"; (b) the inclusion under this heading of various conditions (2) including not only true malignant myelosclerosis as described by Lewis and Szur, but also acute myelodysplasia with myelofibrosis, and cases of acute myeloid leukemia with myelofibrosis which are difficult to classify. The confusion has been increased even more by certain authors (3) who identify megakaryoblastic leukemia with malignant myelosclerosis without reason.

In this paper, we propose to discuss the relations that may exist between the different syndromes, after reviewing the diagnostic criteria for acute myelodysplasia with myelofibrosis (AMF), in the light of our observation of 10 patients with AMF studied over the past few years at the Henri Mondor

Hospital in parallel with large number of patients with other conditions that are associated with marrow fibrosis.

PATIENTS AND METHODS

For this study, we reviewed the files of the patients referred to the Central Service of Hematology of the Henri Mondor Hospital for pancytopenia of sudden onset and whose bone marrow biopsy showed a cellular marrow with myelofibrosis. We included only patients with no known previous history of hemopathology and in whom the above features were the first manifestation of the illness.

A Jamshidi needle was used to obtain all the biopsies, which were then fixed with Bouin's solution, embedded in Histomed (a mixture of paraffin and plastic) and cut in 2-μm sections.

The criteria for inclusion in the study were fullfilled in various conditions, including (a) bony metastases of cancers, Hodgkin's disease, acute lymphoblastic leukemia, lymphoproliferative disorders, and (b) myeloid disorders.

The first group is easily recognizable by the architectural and histomorphological picture of the cell proliferation. However, the myeloid disorders are more difficult to analyze because of their cell polymorphism. Only by bone marrow biopsy is it possible to classify the myeloid disorders into three categories: acute myeloid leukemia with marked myelofibrosis and homogeneous cell proliferation, malignant myelosclerosis, and acute myelodysplasia with myelofibrosis (AMF).

In 1981, we published eight cases of AMF (4): subsequently two further cases satisfying the same criteria have been added to the group.

RESULTS

The AMF was idiopathic in half of the cases (Table 1), four men and one woman, aged over 50 years. In the other five cases, the AMF was secondary to chemotherapy and/or radiotherapy given for nonhematological conditions. These five patients were women between 34 and 71 years of age. In all 10 cases, the absence of organomegaly was noted. Normochromic normocytic anemia was present in all but one case (case 4). Absolute reticulocyte counts were found to be low in the six cases in which they were determined (Table 2). All cases showed abnormalities of red cell morphology, including anisocytosis, poikilocytosis, polychromasia, macrocytosis, and in some cases schizocytosis and occasional tear-drop cells. Neutropenia and thrombocytopenia were always present, the latter ranging from 10 to 96 $\times$ 10^9/liter; leukopenia

Table 1 Clinical Features in AMF

Number	Sex	Age (Years)	Primary Disease	Previous Therapy[a]	Status[a] (Months)	Evolution to Overt Leukemia
1	M	67			D (3)	No
2	F	77			D (3)	No
3	M	72			D (6)	No
4	M	55			D (7)	No
5	M	53			D (12)	Yes
6	F	58	Breast carcinoma	C	D (9)	No
7	F	71	Ovarian carcinoma	C	D (10)	Yes
8	F	37	Multiple sclerosis	C	D (12)	Yes
9	F	34	Melanoma	C	D (10)	Yes
10	F	64	Breast carcinoma	C + R	A (5)	No

[a]C = chemotherapy; R = radiotherapy; A = alive; D = died.

was found in all but case 8. A leukoerythroblastic picture was observed in three cases. Examination of several smears showed the presence of rare blast cells, the majority of which showed no peroxidase activity (cases 1, 2, 3, 8).

The bone marrow aspirates (Table 3) gave a dry tape in four cases but was analyzable in six cases. The cellularity was decreased in all but case 10. Morphological abnormalities of the myeloid lines were identical to those found in refractory anemia with excess of blasts (RAEB) and/or RAEB-T (5). An excess of immature cells of the granulocytic series, as well as dysgranulopoiesis were always present, as was dyserythropoiesis with a variable percentage of ringed sideroblasts. On bone marrow smears, the rare megakaryocytes were dystrophic, of micromegakaryocytic type. Blast cells were also seen, some of which closely resembled megakaryoblasts.

An electron microscope examination of the marrow was done in two instances (cases 4 and 8). In both cases, the blast population was found to be polymorphic, consisting of immature erythroblasts (recognizable by the presence of rhopheocytic vesicles and fine deposits of iron in the mitochondria), myeloblasts (containing rare peroxidase-positive granules), and cells of the megakaryocyte series [identified by the platelet peroxidase (PPO) reaction] (6) (Fig. 1).

The cells were found to be heterogeneous in all the biopsies, which appeared very similar for all cases (Figs. 2 and 3). Bone marrow cellularity was

Table 2 Peripheral Blood Findings in AMF

	Patient's Number									
Component	1	2	3	4	5	6	7	8	9	10
Hemoglobin (g/dl)	5.7	6.6	7.4	8	5.4	8.8	6.7	6.7	10.8	8.6
MCV (fl)	94	89	96	102	94	80	88	71	92	81
Reticulocyte ($\times 10^9$/liter)	16	ND	29	ND	ND	ND	14	24	0	33
Platelets ($\times 10^9$/liter)	10	13	22	39	68	41	18	42	39	96
White blood cells ($\times 10^9$/liter)	1.5	1.2	2.2	2.7	2.1	1.6	1.2	7.5	0.9	3
Polymorphonuclear leukocytes ($\times 10^9$/liter)	0.1	0.7	1	0.6	0.7	0.4	0.4	1	0.3	0.8
Blasts ($\times 10^9$/liter)	0.6	0.1	0.1	0	0	0	0	0.4	0	0
Leukoerythroblastic	-	-	-	-	-	+	+	+	-	-

ND = Not done.

Table 3 Bone Marrow Smears in Six Patients with AMF

	Patient's Number[a]					
	1	2	4	5	9	10
Cellularity	d	d	d	d	d	n
Blasts (%)	1	1	22	6	12	5
Myeloblasts + promyelocytes (%)	39	21	4	4	8	4
Myelocytes (%)	6	17	11	13	21	5
Metamyelocytes + polymorphonuclears (%)	3	14	14	14	12	1
Erythroblasts (%)	30	27	33	53	5	79
Ring sideroblasts (%)	15	24	9	46	68	6

[a]Cases 3, 6, 7, 8: dry taps. d = Decreased; n = normal.

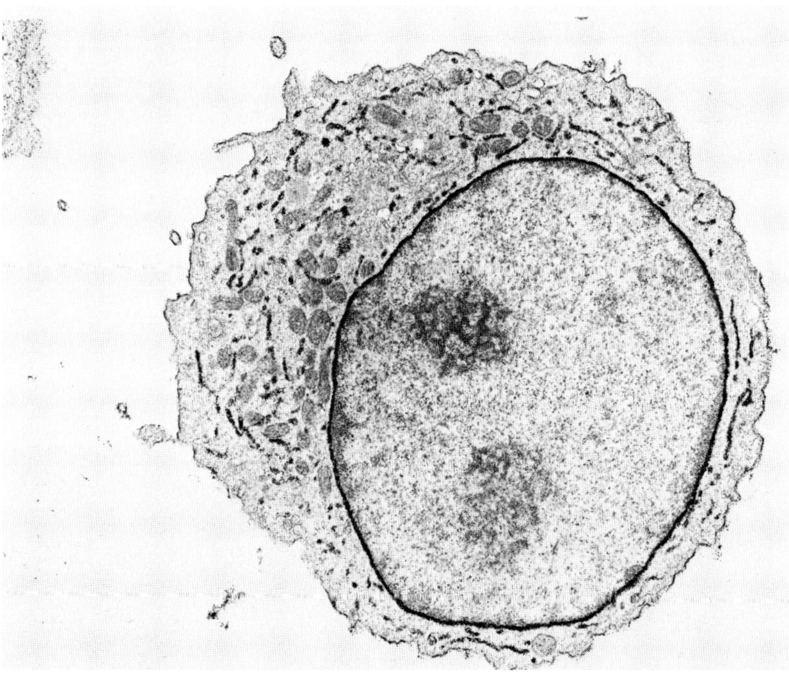

Figure 1 EM of a circulating blast cell identified as a megakaryoblast by the platelet peroxidose reaction (case 7). 7700X.

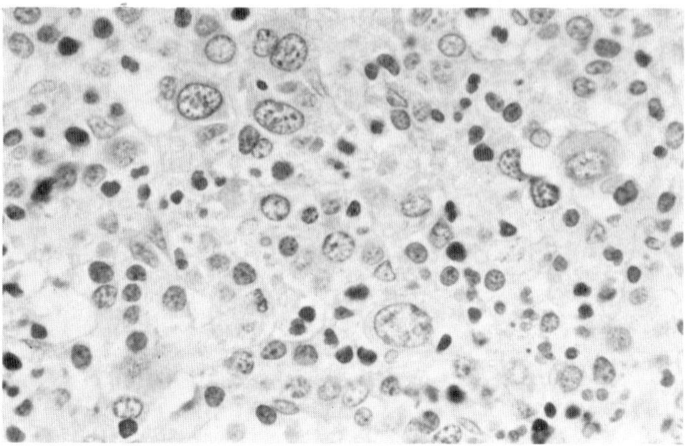

Figure 2 AMF megakaryocytes have poorly lobulated nuclei. They also appear round-shaped. One can recognize clusters of erythroblasts and blast cells difficult to identify (case 7). Hematoxylin & Eosin stain, 500X.

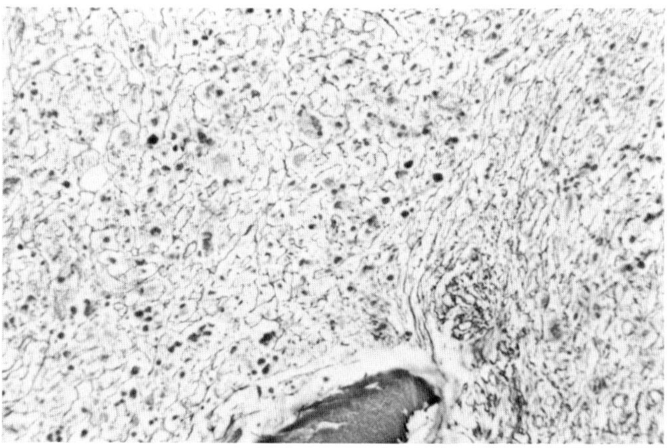

Figure 3 AMF. The reticulin network is diffusely increased without collagen formation. Gomori stain, 300X.

considerably increased and the disappearance of fat cells was noted. Megakaryocytes were numerous, with large regular nuclei with fine chromatin. The nuclei were most often round-shaped rather than lobulated. Cells of the granulocytic series were present, with a definite preponderance of the more immature forms, along with clustered or individual erythroblasts. All samples contained immature cells difficult to identify on histological section. The reticulin network was homogenously dense and collagen tissue was rare or absent. No osteosclerosis was found.

The clinical course varied (Table 1). Of the five idiopathic cases, four patients (cases 1, 2, 3, 4) died of bone marrow failure 2–6 months after onset of symptoms. Patient 5 is alive 12 months after onset of the illness. At present, he is in an acute leukemic phase, with 15×10^9/liter circulating blasts, 20% of which are peroxidase positive. Of the five cases secondary to chemotherapy, three patients died of acute leukemia 4-9 months following the onset of symptoms. One of these (case 7) was an AML/M2 (FAB), while in two cases the acute myeloid leukemia was polymorphic, both by light microscopy (case 9) and electron microscopy (case 8). In the two remaining patients (cases 6 and 10), the bone marrow insufficiency remained stable for 5-9 months. In case 10, blast cells are now appearing in the circulating blood, concurrently with worsening thrombocytopenia.

DISCUSSION

In this report, we have described the hematological findings in 10 cases of acute myelodysplasia with myelofibrosis (AMF). This syndrome is characterized (4) by (a) severe pancytopenia of sudden onset in patients with no previous hematological history, (b) absence of organomegaly, (c) association of reticulin fibrosis, dysmyelopoiesis, and an excess of blast cells of the three myeloid lines, particularly the megakaryocyte series. In half of our patients, the illness occurred following chemotherapy and/or radiotherapy.

AMF must be distinguished from the myelodysplasic syndromes (MDS), malignant myelosclerosis, and megakaryoblastic leukemia.

The myelodysplasic syndromes are myeloid stem cell disorders characterized by qualitative defects of one or more cell lines resulting in peripheral cytopenia in contrast with a marrow that appears cellular on aspiration or biopsy (7, 8). MDS generally occurs in persons over 50 years of age and sometimes precedes the appearance of acute myeloid leukemia. AMF resembles MDS by its marked dysmyelopoiesis. It differs from MDS by its sudden onset and marked myelofibrosis. In MDS, we have found the reticulin network at diagnosis to be normal or slightly increased. The appearance of myelofibrosis is nevertheless possible during the course of acquired sideroblastic anemia (9). Borderline cases between AMF and MDS have been reported (10).

Cases that satisfy the criteria for AMF have been reported under the labels of malignant myelosclerosis and megakaryoblastic leukemia, terms that have tended to be used synonymously in recent publications.

Malignant myelosclerosis has been defined by Lewis and Szur according to the criteria presented above (1). They considered this condition to be an acute form of agnogenic myeloid metaplasia. This interpretation, which they reaffirmed in a more recent report (11), is the basis for the term "malignant myelosclerosis." This condition is extremely rare, and since its initial description only a few strictly identical cases have been reported (12-15). AMF can be distinguished from malignant myelosclerosis by bone marrow biopsy: AMF marrow is more cellular and contains numerous megakaryocytes with large poorly lobulated nuclei with light chromatin, rather than the hyperchromatic nuclei that are distorted by fibrosis in malignant myelosclerosis (Fig. 4).

Megakaryoblastic leukemia is also extremely uncommon (16) and difficult to diagnose because of the following problems: (a) difficulty in recognizing megakaryoblasts as the more immature forms require special technique for demonstration of platelet peroxidase (6), and this is rarely done, (b) marrow fibrosis interferes with bone marrow aspiration and examination. In most cases, the diagnosis is based on the examination of the rare circulating blasts which reflect only indirectly the condition of the bone marrow. Most reported

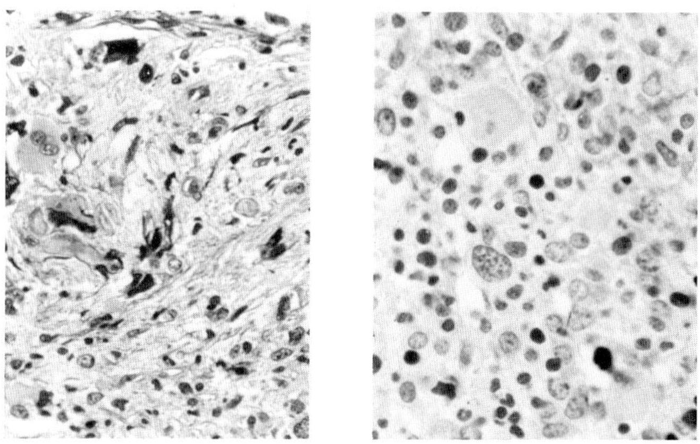

Figure 4 Malignant myelosclerosis (left) and AMF (right). Hematoxylin & Eosin stain, 500X.

cases of megakaryoblastic leukemia do not consist of purely megakaryoblastic proliferations, but rather are polymorphic myeloid disorders in which the involvement of the megakaryocytic series seems to predominate. Certain cases of megakaryoblastic leukemia fulfill the diagnostic criteria for AMF (17, 18). In these cases, we prefer to regard them as AMF, as this underlines the panmyeloid nature of the condition.

It should be noted that in half of our cases the illness occurred following chemotherapy, the interval between therapy and onset ranging from 6 to 60 months. In recent years, many cases of myeloid disorders as complicating drug and/or radiation treatment have been reported. Certain cases present a picture of an acute leukemia with an appearance indistinguishable from a de novo leukemia. In a large proportion of cases, particularly when diagnosed early, variously associated hypoplasia, myelofibrosis, dysmyelopoiesis, and blastic proliferation of several myeloid lines make these conditions difficult to classify in the FAB system (19-22). AMF is set apart by its sudden onset and severe cytopenia. The existence of both AMF secondary to chemotherapy and apparently idiopathic forms might suggest the possibility of a carcinogenic agent as the origin of the so-called primary forms. It should be noted that patient number 3 had been previously subjected to occupational exposure to benzene. Although no exposure to myelotoxic agents could be discovered for the other cases, the retrospective nature of our study does not permit definitive conclusions. Only by a study of a large series of patients would it be feasible to explore the possible role of environmental factors in the etiology of this disease.

REFERENCES

1. Lewis, S. M., and Szur, L. (1963). Malignant myelosclerosis. *Br. Med. J. ii*: 472–476.
2. Bearman, R. M., Pangalis, T. A., and Rappaport, H. (1979). Acute ("malignant") myelosclerosis. *Cancer 43*: 279–293.
3. Chan, W. C., Brynes, R. K., Kim, T. H., Verras, A., Schick, C., Green, R. S., and Ragab, A. H. (1983). Acute megacaryoblastic leukemia in early childhood. *Blood 62*: 92–98.
4. Sultan, C., Sigaux, F., Imbert, M., and Reyes, F. (1981). Acute myelodysplasia with myelofibrosis: a report of eight cases. *Br. J. Haematol. 49*: 11–16.
5. Bennett, J. M., Catovsky, D., Daniel, M. T., Flandrin, G., Galton, D. A. G., Gralnick, H. R., and Sultan, C. (1982). Proposals for the classification of the myelodysplastic syndromes. *Br. J. Haematol. 51*: 189–199.
6. Breton-Gorius, J., Reyes, F., Duhamel, G., Najman, A., and Gorin, N. C.

(1978). Megakaryoblastic acute leukemia: identification by the ultrastructural demonstration of platelet peroxidase. *Blood 51*: 45-60.
7. Sultan, C. (1977). Dysmyelopoietic syndromes, "Classification of acute leukemia." Moderated by H. R. Gralnick. *Ann. Int. Med. 87*: 740-753.
8. Imbert, M., Pierre, R., and Vardiman, J. (1983). In *Hematology*. Education program of the American Society of Hematology, pp. 1-5.
9. Yeung, K. Y., and Trowbridge, A. A. (1977). Idiopathic acquired sideroblastic anemia terminating in acute myelofibrosis. *Cancer 39*: 359-365.
10. Imbert, M., Jarry, M. T., Tulliez, M., and Breton-Gorius, J. (1983). Platelet peroxidase deficiency in a case of myelodysplastic syndrome with myelofibrosis. *J. Clin. Pathol. 36*: 1223-1228.
11. Lewis, S. M., and Szur, L. (1974). Today's treatment. Blood and neoplastic diseases. *Br. Med. J. 4*: 399-602.
12. Castleman, B., Mc Neely, B. V., eds. (1966). Case records of the Massachusetts General Hospital (case 24-1966). *N. Engl. J. Med. 274*: 1200-1208.
13. Bird, T., and Proctor, S. J. (1977). Malignant myelosclerosis. Myeloproliferative disorder or leukemia? *Am. J. Clin. Pathol. 67*: 512-520.
14. Fabich, D. R., Raich, P. C. (1977). Acute myelofibrosis. A report of three cases. *Am. J. Clin. Pathol. 67*: 334-338.
15. Lefevre, P., Ricard, M. F., Imbert, M., Reyes, F., Pinaudeau, Y., and Sultan, C. (1979). La myelofibrose maligne. Une observation. *Nouvelle Presse Médicale 8*: 3545-3567.
16. Flandrin, G., Daniel, M. T., Valensi, F., Schaison, G., and Breton-Gorius, J. (1977). Leucémie aigue à mégacaryoblastes: Etude clinique et morphologique de 11 observations. *Act. Hématol. 11*: 200-212.
17. Den Ottolander, G. J., Te Velde, J., Brederoo, P., Graedts, J. P., Slee, P. H. I., Willenze, R., Zwaan, F. E., Haak, H. L., Muller, H., and Bieger, R. (1979). Megakaryoblastic leukaemia (acute myelofibrosis). A report of three cases. *Br. J. Haematol. 42*: 9-20.
18. Bain, B. J., Catovsky, D., O'Brien, M., Prentice, H. T., Lawlor, E., Kumaran, T. O., Mc Cann, S. R., Matutes, E., and Galton, D. A. G. (1981). Megakaryoblastic leukemia presenting as acute myelofibrosis. A study of four cases with the platelet-peroxydase reaction. *Blood 58*: 206-213.
19. Bennett, J. M., Catovsky, D., Daniel, M. T., Flandrin, G., Galton, D. A. G., Gralnick, H. R., and Sultan, C. (1976). Proposals for the classification of the acute leukaemias. *Br. J. Haematol. 33*: 451-458.
20. Foucar, K., Mc Kenna, R. W., Bloomfield, C. D., Bowers, T. K., and Brunning, R. D. (1979). Therapy related leukemia. A panmyelosis. *Cancer 43*: 1285-1296.
21. Berger, R., Bernheim, A., Daniel, M. T., Valensi, F., and Flandrin, G. (1981). Karyotype and cell phenotypes in acute leukemia following other diseases. *Blood Cells 7*: 287-292.
22. Groupe Français de Cytogenetique Hematologique. (1984). Chromosome analysis of 63 cases of secondary non lymphoid blood disorders. A co-operative study. *Cancer Genet. Cytogenet. 12*: 95-104.

9

Cytogenetic Studies in Myelofibrosis and Related Conditions

SYLVIA D. LAWLER AND G. JOHN SWANSBURY
Royal Marsden Hospital, London, England

INTRODUCTION

Historical Perspective

During the last two decades, the results of cytogenetic research have led to an appreciation, by both scientists and clinicians, of the importance of nonrandom chromosomal abnormalities in malignant and premalignant diseases, particularly those involving the hematopoietic system.

The first human nonrandom clonal chromosomal abnormality to be associated with a particular malignancy, chronic myeloid leukemia (CML), was the Philadelphia chromosome (Ph^1), discovered by Nowell and Hungerford in 1960 (1). The expectation that specific chromosomal abnormalities would be found in other malignant disorders was not realized until the 1970s when, after the discovery that the Ph^1 chromosome arose from a translocation between the long arms of chromosomes 9 and 22 (2), other specific translocations were described in acute leukemias and a lymphoma of defined cell type. Thus, acute promyelocytic leukemia (FAB type M3) is associated with a translocation between the long arms of chromosomes 15 and 17, and acute myeloid leukemia (AML) of M2 type with a translocation between the long arms of chromosomes 8 and 21, whereas a translocation between the long arms of chromosomes 8 and 14 is specific for Burkitt's lymphoma (reviewed in Ref. 3).

Although such specific karyotypic abnormalities are not found in all types of hematologic disorders, the involvement of particular chromosomes in losses, gains, or structural rearrangements is not a random process. For example, the presence of an extra number 8 chromosome is a feature of various chronic and acute hematologic disorders and loss of number 7 occurs in about 4% of cases of AML (4); other chromosomes, e.g., numbers 2, 3, 4, 10, and 18, are rarely involved.

During the 1980s, it became apparent that some of the specific rearrangements involved chromosomes that carried cellular oncogenes and that the breakpoints were in the vicinity of the sites of the oncogenes. For example, in Ph^1-positive CML the c-*abl* gene (cellular homolog of the Abelson murine leukemia virus) is translocated from chromosome 9 to chromosome 22 and, concomitantly, the c-*sis* gene (cellular homolog of the simian sarcoma virus) is translocated from chromosome 22 to chromosome 9 (5, 6). It seems likely that alteration in structure or genomic position, or aberrant expression of cellular oncogenes, is involved in tumorigenesis.

No specific chromosomal abnormality has yet been associated with myelofibrosis (MF). In our review of the cytogenetics of MF, we have investigated the data for the occurrence of nonrandom chromosomal changes peculiar to this disorder.

General Hematological Applications of Cytogenetic Studies

Chromosomal findings have both diagnostic and prognostic implications in a variety of hematologic disorders (3). For example, in CML, the importance of distinguishing between Ph^1-positive and Ph^1-negative patients is generally accepted. The Ph^1-negative patients, with either apparently normal chromosomes or abnormalities other than the Ph^1, have a poorer prognosis than the Ph^1-positive patients, due to deaths occurring within the first year after diagnosis.

Follow-up cytogenetic studies are valuable because changes in chromosomal status can often be related to changes in the patient's clinical condition. In patients with a normal karyotype in the cells of the marrow at diagnosis, abnormalities may arise when a previously chronic condition evolves into an acute phase. Alternatively, chromosomally abnormal clones detected at diagnosis may develop further abnormalities during the course of the disease, and this may also be associated with an acceleration of the disease process.

TECHNICAL CONSIDERATIONS

Cytogenetic Divide Between Banding and Nonbanding

In assessing cytogenetic studies, it is necessary to distinguish between the "banding" and "prebanding" eras. Until 1970, the 23 human chromosome pairs were defined according to their length and the position of their centromere. This meant that because of similarity in size, some chromosomes could only be identified as members of one of seven groups (labeled A to G) with similar morphology and that only those rearrangements involving gross changes in chromosome size could be detected. The development of techniques pioneered by Caspersson et al. (7) has allowed each pair of chromosomes to be distinguished by a distinct banding pattern.

In our review of the published cases of myelofibrosis, we have included only those cases where banding methods were attempted, even if the poor morphology of the chromosomes made complete analysis impossible. The results of prebanding studies are summarized in the next section, Summary of Main Points of Prebanding Studies.

Tissues Used for Study

In studying the cytogenetics of most hematologic disorders, the tissue of choice is bone marrow. In myelofibrosis, however, bone marrow aspiration frequently fails to provide adequate material. When there are extramedullary hematopoietic cells, other tissues may give a satisfactory result. In particular, blood samples are used, both for ease of access and because 24-hr unstimulated cultures do yield dividing cells in a proportion of cases. It must be appreciated, however, that metaphases with a normal karyotype, detected in unstimulated blood cultures, could represent reactive cells of the lymphoid series.

Hematopoietic cells obtained from trephines (8) have also been used and clones have been detected in cultures from a lymph node infiltrated with granulocytes (9). Cells derived from spleen biopsy can be used: however, studies on several different tissues are recommended since blast cells in different sites may derive from largely separate populations of hematopoietic cells. Brandt et al. (10) reported a case in which an abnormal clone was detected in bone marrow but not spleen. This is the reverse to findings in some studies of CML, which demonstrated the splenic origin of blast crisis (10a).

No abnormal clones have been detected in marrow-derived fibroblasts and such cells are considered to be inappropriate for cytogenetic study (see below).

Cytogenetic Nomenclature

Description of chromosomes follows the ISCN conventions (11); a few relevant points are summarized here:

The human chromosome complement, the karyotype, is normally 22 homologous pairs (autosomes), described by a number that in general corresponds to decreasing order of size, plus two further "sex" chromosomes, XX in the female and XY in the male.

The longer and shorter arms of chromosomes are referred to by the letters p and q, respectively.

A chromosomal abnormality is described as constitutional when it has been present from birth. It is, in most cases, present in all the tissues of the body. In addition, a small proportion of cells have abnormalities that arise spontaneously, probably as a result of errors in chromosome replication or dysjunction subsequent to damage by radiation or chemicals.

It is implicit that other chromosomal abnormalities are acquired as part of a neoplastic process: these are usually considered to arise from a single cell and are described as clonal, a clone being a population of cells with the same or related chromosomal abnormalities. Only gross rearrangements of the karyotype can be detected by light microscopy, so absence of chromosome abnormality cannot be taken to imply that the cell is therefore functionally normal.

Deletion of a chromosome describes loss of part of it and is indicated by a - following the chromosome number (e.g., 5q- indicates a chromosome number 5 that is missing part of its long arms). A + after the number indicates a net gain in chromosome size as a result of translocation. An abnormal chromosome whose origin cannot be determined is described as a marker (mar).

Loss of a whole chromosome is referred to as monosomy, gain as trisomy. These are indicated by - and + before the chromosome number. A cell with 46 chromosomes is diploid; aneuploidy refers to a cell with other than 46 chromosomes.

For the purposes of this review, a clone is defined as at least two cells with the same structural change or with the same extra chromosome or at least three cells with the same chromosome lost. Any case with a clone according to these criteria has been included. If a clone was present, then the finding of one cell with a normal karyotype was taken to indicate the presence of a population of normal cells. If no clone was detected then at least five cells had to be fully analyzed for the case to be included here as having a normal karyotype.

A clone has been described as complex in this text if more than two chromosomes were involved.

SUMMARY OF MAIN POINTS OF PREBANDING STUDIES

Although for our analysis cases are excluded if there was no information on banded karyotypes, much work had already been done in this group of myeloid disorders before the advent of the banding era. The findings before banding, and in the early years of the application of this technique, have been well reviewed by Sandberg (12).

Until 1978, Sandberg (12) found that in myeloid metaplasia, including diseases described as myelofibrosis, panmyelosis, and marrow dysplasia, over 50% of the cases did not have any chromosomal abnormalities. He pointed out that the majority of the cases with normal karyotypes were contributed by a small number of laboratories and that the apparent proportion of chromosomally abnormal cases was too large because chromosomally normal cases were less likely to be reported. This may be true also of subsequent reports.

Sandberg commented on the fact that in many of these cases the abnormal clone did not constitute the whole of the cell population, chromosomally normal cells being in the majority, and that the proportion of clonal cells present did not appear to correlate with prognosis.

SUMMARY OF LITERATURE

Ascertainment

The papers reviewed here were found using Medline (a computer-assisted search of details prepared from *Index Medicus*), augmented by a personal survey of the literature.

What Has Been Accepted as Myelofibrosis

Myelofibrosis has diffuse boundaries of definition with consequent variety of nomenclature. Furthermore, many reports have given insufficient hematologic detail for us to attempt reclassification. Therefore, for this review, cases reported to have "myelofibrosis" have been accepted without querying the diagnoses, which have been grouped as follows:

1. PMF
   a. Primary (chronic) myelofibrosis

   b. Agnogenic myeloid metaplasia
   c. Myelosclerosis
   d. Undifferentiated myeloproliferative disorder
2. AMF
   a. Acute myelofibrosis
   b. Acute agnogenic myeloid metaplasia
   c. Acute megakaryoblastic leukemia
   d. Malignant myelosclerosis
3. SMF
   a. Secondary myelofibrosis

The abbreviations PMF, AMF, and SMF, or the first name in each group, will be used to include the others, unless otherwise indicated.

Primary myelofibrosis involving less than one-third of the marrow has been classified as undifferentiated myeloproliferative disorder (UMPD) by some authors (13), as a condition distinct from that with greater than one-third. However, it has been shown that having a marrow with fibrosis of either less or more than one-third does not have a significant effect on prognosis (14): hence the inclusion here of UMPD in group 1. Furthermore, many authors have not given details of the marrow histology, so it seemed inappropriate to try to distinguish between MF and UMPD.

Fifty-five cases of PMF in which an abnormal clone was detected are listed in Table 1. Thirty-six cases that had apparently normal karyotypes are not tabulated, including two with only normal chromosomes found on initial study and in whom chromosomally abnormal clones were detected after they had developed leukemia (cases 3 and 6 of Ref. 15).

All the cases of AMF and myelofibrosis secondary to polycythemia rubra vera (PRV), CML, and other disorders are listed in Tables 2-5, respectively.

In the tables, the letters RMH indicate cases with previously unpublished details that were studied at the Royal Marsden Hospital.

Chromosome Findings in Chronic and Acute Myelofibrosis

An indication of the frequency of structural and numerical involvement of different chromosomes in the clones detected in PMF and AMF is given in Figures 1, a and b, the details being derived from Tables 1 and 2.

The following is a commentary of some of the features apparent in the Figures:

1. Chromosome 1 is commonly involved in translocations in various hematopoietic disorders (16), including MF. In at least 8 of the 14 cases here,

Table 1 Cases of PMF with a Chromosomally Abnormal Clone

Case	Ref	I/D	Sex	Age	Subsequent Diagnosis	State	Survival (Months)	Tissue	Number of Cells Analyzed	Percent Abnormal	Clonal Karyotype
2	13	367	M	45		Dead	37	PB+BM	nk	95	45,XY,−1,−7,+t(1p−;4q;7q),4q−
3	13	386	M	62		Dead	1	Blood	nk	100	45,XY,−C (?7−9)
4	13	414	F	74		Alive	27	Blood	nk	65	47,XX,+?20q−,18p+
5	13	418	F	72		Dead	66	Blood	nk	25	46,XX,1q+,1q−
21	52	532	M	nk		Alive	9	nk	nk	nk	50,XY,+1p−,+8,+9,+21
24	32	225	F	70		nk	nk	Blood	39	97	46,XX,7q−,−9,+mar
27	9	single case	F	54	AML	Dead	7	PB+BM	91	61	49,XX,+"G",+C,t(1q?;?),+19
28	56	case 1		nk		nk	nk	Marrow	nk	100	47,X?,+9
29	56	case 2		nk		nk	nk	Marrow	nk	100	47,X?,+9
30	49	single case[a]	F	59		Alive	13	Marrow	290	100	47,X,del(X)(q22),+del(X)(q22)
31	32	87	M	nk		nk	nk	Marrow	85	20	45,X,−Y
32	32	case 166	F	nk		nk	nk	Marrow	83	60	47,XX,+8
33	32	230	M	nk		nk	nk	Marrow	90	100	45,X,−Y
34	32	326	M	nk		nk	nk	Marrow	50	100	49,X,−Y,+mars(?dicY)
35	32	338	M	nk		nk	nk	Marrow	51	12	47,XY,+8
37	57	single case	F	50		Alive	65	PB+BM	40	100	46,XX,del(20)(q11)
38	58	KMN	M	70		Dead	66	Blood	20	100	46,XY,del(20)(q11)
40	17	EJ	F	38		Alive	204	Blood	40	100	46,XX,−6,+t(1;6)(q25;p22)
42	59	DG	F	64		Dead	6	Marrow	19	nk	47,XX,+13
43	60	single case	M	47	AML	Dead	136	Marrow	23	100	46,XY,−6,+t(1;6)(q23;p21)
46	61	AB	M	40		Dead	11	Blood	10	100	46,XY,−7,+t(1;7)(p1?;p11), t(17;?)(p;?)

Table 1 (Continued)

Case	Ref	I/D	Sex	Age	Subsequent Diagnosis	State	Survival (Months)	Tissue	Number of Cells Analyzed	Percent Abnormal	Clonal Karyotype
47	62	case 1	F	75		nk	nk	Blood	4	75	47,XX,+8,+9 and has constitutional t(13;14)
48	55	case 1	M	10		Dead	24	Blood	31	100	45,XY,–7
56	46	DM	F	70		nk	3	Blood	nk	nk	47,XX,+8
58	63	case 5	M	53		nk	nk	Blood	nk	nk	46,XY,–12,+der(12)t(1;12)(q11;q24)
59	64	single case VH	M	23		Dead	nk	Blood	30	100	47,X,–Y,+18q–,+18q–,+C,–F
61	43	EC	F	61		Dead	72	PB+BM	nk	100	47,XX,+1q–,t(1;2)(q1?;q1?),22q–,t(6;7),+r
62	26	Pt. 12, Table 1	F	78		nk	nk	nk	nk	73	46,XX,del(15)(q14–q23?)
64	49	3	F	70		Alive	144	Blood	nk	100	46,XX,13q–
66	19	case 4	F	nk	AML	nk	42	Marrow	nk	nk	47,XX,+21,5q–
68	65	case 10 DO	M	53	AML	Dead	24	nk	nk	nk	45,XY,–C ?
69	65	case 13 EM	M	71	AML	Dead	44	nk	nk	nk	47,XY,+C
70	65	case 14 SG	M	65	AML	Dead	77	nk	nk	nk	?,XY,Ph^1 +ve, aneuploidy.
76	29	case 5	M	69		Dead	12	Blood	11	64	47,XXY(Constitutional),20q–
77	40	case 1	F	2		Dead	2	Blood	33	100	50,XX,+21 (Constitutional),+8,+19,+19/+8,+21

78	66	single case	M	14		Dead	92	PB+BM	50	100	48,XY,+8,+21
82	67	case 21	F	28	AML	nk	nk	nk	34	100	46,XX,t(9;22)
84	68	single case	M	55		Dead	144	Blood	39	100	46,XY,dup(1q)
88	15	case 4	F	19	AUL	Dead	9	nk	nk	100	47,XX,+21.
91	15	case 11	F	49		Dead	60	PB+BM	nk	80	47,XX,+16
94	15	case 14	M	56		Alive	30	Spleen	nk	11	47,XY,+21
98	15	case 18	M	46		Alive	9	nk	nk	25	46,XY,–8,+t(1q;2q),inv(13),i17q
99	15	case 19	F	33		Alive	96	nk	nk	6	46,XX,–12,+t(5;12)(q14;q13)
106	RMH	Chpl	F	71		Alive	50	Marrow	9	nk	48,XX,+6,+20
112	42	case 26	F	nk		nk	nk	PB+BM	46	100	46,XX,12p–
113	42	case 27	F	nk		nk	nk	Blood	75	99	47,XX,–20,5q–,11q–,+mar,+mar
115	42	case 31	F	nk		nk	nk	Blood	39	74	46,XX,18p+
116	42	case 32	F	nk		nk	nk	PB+BM	13	100	46,XX,13q–
117	42	case 36	M	nk		nk	nk	Blood	13	61	46,XY,9q–
118	42	case 37		nk		nk	nk	PB+BM	23	100	46,XX,–15,5q–,7q+,13q–,+mar
120	42	case 39	M	nk		nk	nk	Blood	nk	nk	46,XY,13q–
124	69	case 1	F	45		nk	nk	Blood	55	100	46,XX,dup(1)(q21–q32)
126	70	single case	F	36		Alive	240	PB+BM	15	100	46,XX,del(11)(q13–q21)
130	RMH	Nea	F	44		Dead	17	Blood	10	100	Complex 5q–
140	10	single case	M	62		Dead	65	BM+Spleen	40	42	47,XY,+mar

[a]Previously had multiple sclerosis.
nk = Not known.

Table 2 All Cases of AMF

Case	Ref	I/D	Sex	Age	Subsequent Diagnosis	State	Survival (Months)	Tissue	Number of Cells Analyzed	Percent Abnormal	Karyotype
8	13	case 342	F	18		Dead	24	Blood	nk	90	47,XX,+8
9	13	case 449	F	27		Alive	13	Blood	nk	95	47,XX,+8
20	52	case 509	M	69		Dead	nk	nk	nk	nk	45,XY,–C,–C,+mar,t(3q–,3q–)
22	71	single case	F	37		Dead	3	Blood	26	54	47,XX,+8 / 45,X,–X
25	72	SH	F	26	AMkL	Dead	5	Blood	25	100	47,XX,+10
26	45	single case[a]	M	78		Dead	1	Blood	7	100	46,XY,–5,t(1p;13q),3p–,t(16q;16q), inv(7),+mar
74	73	single case	M	59	CML	Alive	36	PB+BM	nk	50	47,XY,+8 / 46,XY,t(1;4)(p32;q35)
80	47	case 538	F	2	AML	Dead	nk	Blood	nk	nk	47,XX,–21,+i(21q),+i(21q)
81	47	case 563	M	1	AML	Dead	nk	Blood	nk	nk	50,XY,–1,–B,+C,+C,+1q,+1q,+?D, +19
93	72	BL	F	45	AMkL	Dead	3	Blood	17	0	46,XX
96	72	AD	M	55	AMkL	Dead	7	Blood	nk	0	46,XY

[a]Previously had squamous carcinoma of skin.
nk = Not known; AMkL = acute megakaryoblastic leukemia.

Table 3 All Cases of MF Secondary to PRV

Case	Ref	I/D	Sex	Age	Subsequent Diagnosis	State	Survival (Months)	Tissue	Number of Cells Analyzed	Percent Abnormal	Karyotype
7	13	case 422	F	62		Dead	48	Blood	nk	90	47,XX,+t(1q;1p),t(1q;1p),7q–, 20q–
36	32	WB	M	42	AML	Dead	18	Marrow	44	25	46,XY,t(9;22)
41	17	AS	M	49		Alive	18	Marrow	11	100	46,XY,–13,+t(1;13)(q12;p12)
44	61	FK	M	60		Dead	nk	Blood	15	100	47,XY,–7,+21,+t(1;7)(p1?;p11)
45	61	LW	F	69		Dead	nk	Blood	20	100	46,XX,–7,+t(1;7)(p1?;p11)
57	26	case 2	F	56		Alive	24	PB+BM	103	38	46,XX,del(13)(q11–q22)
60	74	single case	F	53		Dead	12	Blood	121	95	51,XX,+1,+6,+9,+11,–19,+20,+mar, del(2)(q33),20q+.
63	49	case 2	M	62		Alive	48	Blood	13	61	46,XY,9q–
65	65	case 2 BE	F	55	AMML	Dead	36	nk	nk	0	46,XX
92	RMH	Han	F	64		Dead	38	Marrow	10	0	46,XX
101	75	case 2	F	55	AML	Dead	5	Blood	nk	76	51,XX,+t(1;5)(p1?;q1?),t(2;11) (p13;q21),+3,+8,+?8,+C,–15,16p–, +19
102	RMH	Wig	F	72		Alive	14	Marrow	13	0	46,XX
103	RMH	Sci	M	52		nk	nk	Marrow	5	0	46,XY
108	RMH	Fre	F	59		nk	nk	nk	18	0	46,XX
125	76	case 7 LF	F	46	EL	Dead	24	PB+BM	10	100	46,XX,t(6;22)(q27?;q11),–21,+mar later: t(3q+;3q–),–7,+mar
128	RMH	Cha	M	71		Alive	26	Marrow	nk	nk	46,XY,del(20)(q)/44,XY,–6,–21, 5q–,16p+q+,17q+
134	RMH	Sha	M	nk		Alive	98	Marrow	17	0	46,XY

nk = Not known; AMML = acute myelomonocytic leukemia; EL = erythroleukemia.

Table 4 All Cases of MF Secondary to CML

Case	Ref	I/D	Sex	Age	State	Survival (Months)	Tissue	Number of Cells Analyzed	Percent Abnormal	Karyotype
39	58	SEP	M	46	Dead	11	nk	55	100	46,XY,t(9;22),i17q,20q–.
90	RMH	Mor	F	32	Dead	3	Marrow	17	100	46,XX,t(9;22)
127	RMH	Bor	M	28	Dead	11	Marrow	25	100	46,XY,t(9;22)
129	RMH	Dil	F	42	Dead	3	Blood	15	100	46,XX,t(9;22)
131	RMH	Ald	M	43	Dead	1	Marrow	35	100	46,XY,t(9;22),del(7)(p12),–21,+mar
132	RMH	Coo	M	61	Dead	6	PB+BM	58	66	47,XY,+8,t(9;22)
136	RMH	Ram	M	31	Alive	13	Marrow	15	100	46,XY,t(9;22),t(17;20)(p?;q?)
137	RMH	Bur	F	33	Dead	4	Marrow	10	70	46,XX,t(9;22)
138	RMH	Fox	F	52	Dead	6	Marrow	7	100	46,XX,t(9;22)
139	RMH	Mur	F	36	Dead	7	Marrow	12	100	46,XX,t(9;22)

nk = Not known.

Table 5 All Cases of MF Secondary to a Malignancy Other Than PRV or CML

Case	Ref	I/D	Sex	Age	Previous Diagnosis	State	Survival (Months)	Tissue	Number of Cells Analyzed	Percent Abnormal	Karyotype
6	13	case 432	M	56	Ca. prostate	Dead	3	Blood	nk	75	44,XY,−5,−7,−11,+t(7p;12q), t(7p;12q),t(17p,18p),+mars
23	32	case 172	M	49	AML	nk	nk	Blood	39	100	45,X,−Y
52	32	case 281	M	60	AML	nk	nk	Blood	34	0	46,XY
55	32	case 325	F	66	AML	nk	nk	Blood	43	0	46,XX
95	15	case 15	F	62	Ca. Colon	Alive	19	PB+BM	nk	100	46,XX,8q−
97	15	case 17	F	43	HD	Alive	96	nk	nk	100	46,X,Xp−q−,5q−,13q+,15q−
133	RMH	Nai	F	39	HD	Dead	120	Marrow	25	60	46,XX,dup(1)(q21−q32)
135	20	Case 3 JK	M	2	MPD	Dead	4	Marrow	nk	100	45,XY,−7/46,XX,−7,+mar

nk = Not known; HD = Hodgkin's disease.

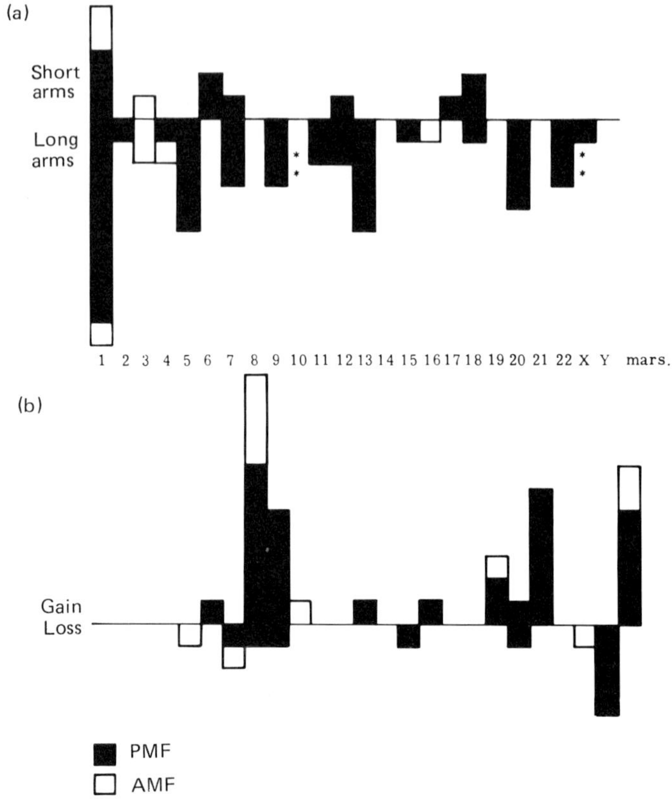

Figure 1 Frequency of involvement of chromosomes in (a) structural change and (b) numerical change. Not included are one case each of iso17q, iso21q and inv7. The asterisks indicate two cases with the Ph[1] translocation, t(9;22).

the result was a net gain in the proximal part of the long arms, a feature that has already been remarked upon (17,16).

Two very similar translocations, t(1;6)(q25;p22) and t(1;6)(q23;p21) occurred in cases 40 and 43 (Table 1). Another translocation involving chromosome 1, t(1;7)(p1?;p11) case 46, was also found in MF secondary to PRV (Table 3, cases 44 and 45). The reporting of further cases is required before an association of particular translocations of chromosome 1 with myelofibrosis can be established.

2. Deletion of part of the long arm of chromosome 5 was observed in four cases of PMF (cases 66, 113, 118, and 130), some other chromosomal abnormality also being present in all. This deletion as the only abnormality has been linked with refractory anemia (18), but it also occurs in other hematopoietic disorders (19), particularly concurrent with other chromosomal abnormalities.

3. Monosomy 7 was reported by Sandberg (12) as being common in MF, but we find only one instance in PMF and none in AMF of the cases scored here. However, two further cases of PMF and three of AMF had a clone marked by loss of a C-group chromosome and the missing chromosome may well have been a 7 in some of these. Among other hematopoietic disorders, monosomy 7 is associated with secondary acute leukemia (4) and a well-defined childhood myeloproliferative disorder (20). Deletion of 7q, common in acute leukemia and particularly secondary acute leukemia, was observed here in only one case of PMF.

4. Trisomy 8 is common in many hematopoietic disorders and occurs here at a notably high frequency in AMF. Completely absent from the reports of PMF and AMF are any of the translocations involving chromosome 8 that are associated with particular types of leukemia, vis. t(8;21) in M2 (21) and t(8;14) in Burkitt's lymphoma (22).

5. Four cases of trisomy 9 were found; this may indicate an association with MF since it is not a frequent occurrence in other hematopoietic disorders. A further case with +9 as part of a complex clone has been reported (23) but has not been included in this review, as cytogenetic studies were performed only after the patient had progressed to acute megakaryoblastic leukemia.

6. Deletion of part of 11q has been linked with acute nonlymphocytic leukemia FAB type M5 (24). However, the breakpoints appear to be different from those of the two cases found here.

7. There are five cases here with abnormality of the long arms of chromosome 13, four being a deletion. Deletions of the long arms of D-group chromosomes had been noted in prebanding studies (25) and the possibility of this particular abnormality being associated with PMF has already been considered (26, 27). In addition to the cases listed here are at least some of the cases of 13q- in MF reported in an abstract (27).

8. The association of 20q- with PRV is well established (28): it appeared in two of the 17 cases listed in Table 3. However, it is not exclusive to PRV (29) and it was found in 4 of the 55 cases of PMF with clones listed in Table 1.

9. Trisomy 21 is a common nonspecific finding in acute leukemias, particularly acute lymphoblastic leukemia (ALL) (30).

10. The Ph^1 chromosome is not exclusive to CML, being also found, rarely, in ALL, AML, and other hematopoietic disorders (31). Thus, its appearance in a case of PMF does not necessarily mean that the diagnosis must be CML. Two cases are given in Table 1, both progressing to AML. However, differing attitudes to classification, affecting the apparent frequency of the Ph^1 in PMF, are represented by instances of changing diagnosis from MF to atypical CML (32) and defining MF as a subtype of CML (8) on the grounds of discovering the Ph^1 chromosome.

11. Loss of the Y chromosome is sometimes found in the bone marrow cells of patients of advancing age but it also occurs in hematopoietic disorders. Details of age were not given in the reports of the four cases found here, but the number of cells analyzed would seem to support the loss as being clonal.

Chromosome Findings in Secondary Myelofibrosis

Patients who develop myelofibrosis either after or concurrent with some other hematologic disorder are likely to have received chemotherapy and/or radiotherapy: in most cases it would not be possible to distinguish between chromosomal abnormalities present as a result of the previous disorder and/or therapy and those presenting in connection with the myelofibrotic state, especially since in very few reported cases have chromosome studies been undertaken in different phases of disease. The monosomy 7 clone of case 135 (Table 5) was detected during his previous condition and thus cannot be a consequence of the later development of MF.

Myelofibrosis Secondary to Polycythemia (Table 3)

Seventeen cases of PRV developing SMF have been found among the literature and our own material, 8 of which are known to have been treated with ^{32}P. The incidence of chromosomal abnormalities at diagnosis of PRV is 13%, but among treated cases it may be as high as 50% (33). However, in the cases reviewed here the incidence is higher still: 12/17 = 60%. Among this group was one case (number 36) with a Ph^1 chromosome. This is an unusual finding in PRV (34). Case 125 had progression of the clone and case 41 had only normal chromosomes found on an initial study; the clone listed was detected subsequently.

Six of the patients had complex clones and this finding was associated with the development of leukemia in two cases. Two other patients were known to have developed leukemia: one had a Ph^1 chromosome and no abnormality was detected in the other. Thus, the majority of patients with PRV and MF, whose disease evolved into leukemia, had chromosomal abnormalities.

Myelofibrosis Secondary to CML (Table 4)

Myelofibrosis can occur during the evolution of MPD. A study of serial trephine biopsies was made by Clough et al. (35) of 45 Ph^1-positive cases of CML. The patients were classified according to the degree of MF, from no increase in reticulum to dense osteomyelosclerosis. Sixteen of the patients (18%) had collagen fibrosis indistinguishable in appearance from agnogenic myeloid metaplasia. Twelve of the patients with SMF died in blast crisis: the death of one of the patients was attributed to septicemia and MF and two others had drug-induced aplasia. No details of the karyotypes of the cases were given, but as far as we are aware this is the only series of cases of SMF in CML with any cytogenetic information. In Table 4, all but one of the Ph^1-positive cases of CML with MF were studied at the Royal Marsden Hospital.

In this group all had the standard Ph^1 translocation t(9;22)(q34;q21). This finding is not unexpected since unusual translocations occur in only about 10% of cases (36).

Three patients had abnormalities in addition to Ph^1; case no. 132 had an extra number 8 chromosome, a frequent finding in Ph^1-positive CML, and another patient, alive at the time of writing, had a second translocation, t(17;20)(q?;q?). One of the patients who died in an acute phase had an isochromosome of the long arm of chromosome 17, an abnormality associated with blast transformation, and also 20q−, a structural abnormality more usually associated with PRV.

In summary, this group of patients with MF in association with CML does not show any unexpected cytogenetic features, the changes seen having also been described in patients with CML without MF. Therefore, there are no cytogenetic features associated with a predisposition of CML to develop MF evident in these few cases.

Myelofibrosis Secondary to Other Disorders (Table 5)

Cytotoxic therapy or irradiation probably contributed to the marrow fibrosis in the eight cases with miscellaneous previous diagnoses including AML, Hodgkin's disease, and cancers of nonhematopoietic types.

One case of particular interest in this group is number 135, a child whose original diagnosis was MPD characterized by monosomy 7 (20). This rare syndrome is clinically distinguishable from juvenile Ph^1-negative CML and Ph^1-positive CML occurring in children. Acute myeloid leukemia is a likely terminal event, but in case 135 the disease terminated in MF. Within 3 months of development of MF, the blood count rose to 300×10^9/liter but the increase affected cells in all stages of myeloid maturation. Another example of the progression of monosomy 7 in childhood to MF was described by Holden et al. (37). In that case, the missing chromosome was described as a C group and it may be interpreted to be a number 7.

Two of the eight patients in this miscellaneous group had normal bone marrow karyotypes, and in three other cases the karyotypes were complex. So, again, these few cases do not show any particular cytogenetic abnormality to be associated with the development of SMF.

Presence of Concurrent Constitutional Abnormality

Evans (38) described two boys with Down's syndrome who developed acute myelofibrosis when aged 19 and 21 months and they quoted a third case (39) with similar clinical features. On the basis of these observations and the data on leukemia collected by the Manchester Children's Tumour Registry, Evans suggested that there was an increased incidence of acute myelofibrosis in children with Down's syndrome and that the disease may be underdiagnosed because histological examination of the bone marrow is not done.

Two Japanese cases with similar clinical features have been described subsequently (40). Both of these cases had abnormal hyperdiploid clones in the marrow with chromosomes additional to the trisomy 21 expected in Down's syndrome. One of these cases is included in Table 1. The chromosomes additional to the extra 21 were an 8 and two 19s. The second case was a mosaic with two clones, one with one extra G group chromosome and the other with two extra G group chromosomes.

In our survey, we have found two other cases with a constitutional abnormality among 91 with primary MF. Case 47 was a childless Dutch female of 75 years with anemia not responding to iron and vitamin B_{12}. She had a translocation t(13;14) in all cells of both PHA-stimulated and unstimulated cultures. In the unstimulated blood culture, there was a minor clone which had, in addition, extra number 8 and 9 chromosomes.

Case 76 had Klinefelter's syndrome, having an extra X chromosome in the constitutional karyotype. The myeloid cells also showed an acquired abnormality, 20q-.

Constitutional abnormalities occur at a frequency of about 0.58% in the population (41). The frequency here is 4/138 (3.5%) but it is possible that the concurrence of constitutional abnormalities and MF in these four cases is a chance finding, the higher frequency being due to selective reporting.

VALUE OF CHROMOSOME STUDIES IN MYELOFIBROSIS AND RELATED CONDITIONS

Frequency of Abnormal Clones

Owing partly to the difficulty of obtaining metaphases suitable for chromomal analysis, there are relatively few reports of cytogenetic study of PMF: only

91 cases were found for this review. Of these 91 cases, a chromosomally abnormal clone was detected in 55 (= 60%). This may be an overestimate of the proportion of patients with clones, since cases with apparently normal karyotypes are less likely to be reported. Conversely, however, the number of clones detected might increase if unstimulated blood was cultured for various periods in each case (42).

Considering the reports of series of cases, rather than anecdotal reports, the proportion of cases with a clone detected is 8/18 (13), 2/10 (32), and 14/20 (15). Another report, not included in this review because of the lack of cytogenetic details, gives 5/19 (43). The overall proportion from these reports is 29/67 (= 40%). This is high for a hematologic condition that has been described as having no evidence to support a neoplastic etiology (44).

A higher proportion (9/11, 82%) of the reported cases of AMF had a clone (qv. Table 2). This may be associated with the more aggressive nature of this disease.

Chromosomes and the Biology of Myelofibrosis

In only two cases of PMF was mention made of previous exposure to possible carcinogens (Table 1, case 94 and case 3 of Ref. 15). Thus, no conclusion can be drawn about such exposure predisposing to MF (see section on SMF, above).

So far, all reported cytogenetic studies of cultured bone marrow-derived fibroblasts have recorded a normal karyotype, both for PMF (45, 46) and AMF (45, 47). Furthermore, these fibroblasts have been shown to be nonclonal using an enzyme (glucose-6-phosphate dehydrogenase, G6PD) assay in females who are heterozygous at the G6PD gene locus (46). Ruutu et al. (48) have studied the erythroid and granulocyte-monocyte precursors in a case of PMF and a case of MF secondary to PRV. In both cases, the cells of all the colonies examined belonged to a chromosomally abnormal clone, with 13q- and 9q-, respectively (Table 1, case 64, and Table 3, case 63). These observations have led to the conclusion that the marrow fibrosis is secondary, possibly a reactive effect, to a monoclonal hematopoietic stem-cell neoplasm (32, 45, 49, 50).

Chromosomes and the Classification of Myelofibrosis

Many of the chromosomal abnormalities reported so far in MF are those already known to be associated with myeloproliferative disorders. These include rearrangements of chromosome 1, +8, 20q-, +21, and the Ph^1. Also appearing to occur at high frequency were 5q-, +9 and 13q-. These, and other of the abnormalities found in MF, also occur in acute leukemia. As with preleukemic cytopenias, some of the abnormalities associated with particular subtypes of acute myeloid leukemia were not found, e.g., t(8;21), even in the cases of MF that did progress to acute leukemia. However, since the FAB type of most of these acute leukemias secondary to MF has not been reported, the absence of FAB-type-specific translocations may be a consequence of the lack of data rather than a true deficiency.

Rather than cytogenetic studies serving to distinguish the different kinds of MPD, therefore, they underline the close relationship between them. Arguments for the classification of AMF as a form of acute leukemia rather than a myeloproliferative disorder have already been reported (51). The occurrence of some chromosomal abnormalities that are also found in acute leukemia suggests that PMF, too, does not merely predispose to leukemia but should be regarded as early malignant disease in which the neoplastic clone is expanding slowly, in only a few cases becoming clinically recognizable as acute leukemia.

Diagnostic and Prognostic Value of Chromosomal Studies

Unlike the situation in cytopenic disorders (52), Nowell and Finan found no general correlation between cytogenetic result and prognosis in MF. The presence of a chromosomally abnormal clone as such did not generally appear to imply imminent progression to acute leukemia or death from the consequences of the hematopoietic disorder, even when the clone was complex (13).

The presence of a chromosomally abnormal clone has been shown to be negatively correlated with response to treatment with androgens (14), and thus in that study was associated with a poor prognosis.

Of the 138 cases of MF reviewed here, 95 had details of survival reported (included in Tables 1-5), 58 being PMF. The survivals were analyzed using the log rank test of Peto et al. (53).

In PMF the survival of patients with apparently normal chromosomes was very similar to that of all the other patients combined: the simple presence or absence of chromosome abnormality was not associated, from these data, with different survival. When the survivals of all the patients were analyzed, survivals of cases with clones were significantly worse ($p < 0.01$) than those without up to 2 years after diagnosis: thereafter, the difference diminished, becoming nonsignificant before the end of the fourth year. The presence of any normal cells, i.e., less than 100% of metaphases with a clonal abnormality, did not appear to improve the prognosis.

When the clones of PMF cases were analyzed in more detail, it was evident that some abnormalities were associated with longer survival than the patients with normal karyotypes, and others with shorter survival: combining all abnormalities together concealed the differences.

The abnormalities associated with better prognosis were:

1. Simple clone with translocation of chromosome 1
2. Any clone with 5q-
3. Simple clone with trisomy 8
4. 13q-
5. Simple clone with 20q-

The abnormalities associated with worse prognosis were:

1. Ph[1] translocation
2. -7 and 7q-
3. Complex clone, except if 5q- present

Other, rarer, abnormalities were not included.

A log rank analysis of the survivals of patients classified as normal, good prognosis, or bad prognosis resulted in chi square values of 37.07 (all cases) and 11.08 (PMF cases) with 2 degrees of freedom ($p < 0.01$) (qv. Fig. 2). However, because there are few instances of each abnormality, the assignments of some to the better or worse categories may prove to be unfounded when more are reported.

It is also difficult to determine from such few data which are the more significant in combinations of chromosomal abnormalities. Trisomy 8 and translocations of chromosome 1, for example, were associated with a good prognosis only if they were part of a simple clone. Conversely, 5q- occurred as part of a complex clone in all instances, yet the patients had a relatively good prognosis.

This deletion, 5q-, also occurs in other hematologic disorders (19). When present as the only abnormality, it has been linked with refractory anemia (18) and usually indicates a relatively benign condition. As part of a complex clone, it is more common in acute leukemia and preleukemic cytopenia with a high likelihood of progression to acute leukemia, although the prognosis is not always bad (54). In MF the occurrence of 5q- with other abnormalities does not appear to indicate imminent transformation to acute leukemia.

Monosomy 7 is associated with primary and secondary acute nonlymphocytic leukemia (54) and a well-defined childhood condition (20). In preleukemic disorders it is considered to indicate a high likelihood of progressing to

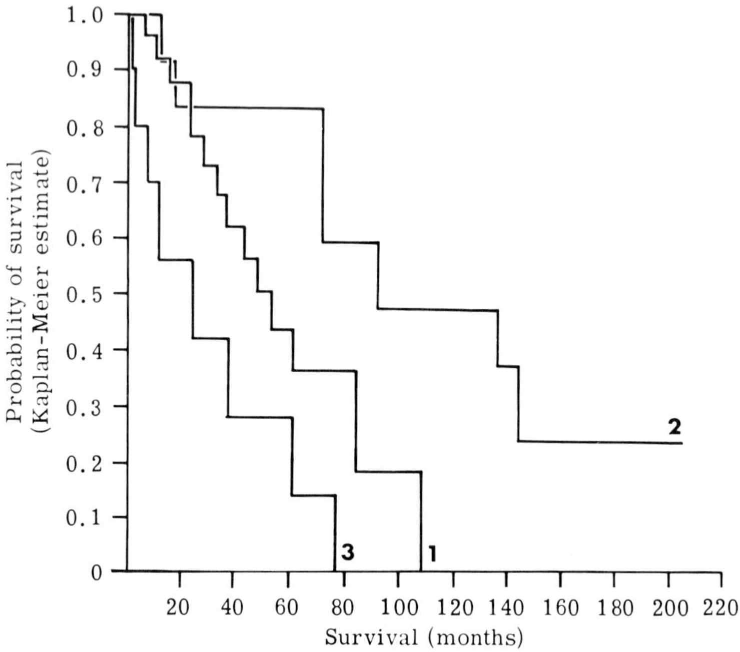

Figure 2 Percent of PMF patients surviving. The classifications are described in the text. 1 = Normal karyotype, 2 = abnormalities associated with better prognosis, 3 = abnormalities associated with worse prognosis.

acute leukemia and although there are few cases discovered in this review, it may be true for MF also (55).

It is concluded that at present no chromosomal abnormality has been discovered that is so highly specific for MF as to be conspicuous in the few cases available for review. Chromosomal abnormalities of the types found in other hematopoietic disorders are also found in MF: these appear to be associated with different prognoses, not always in the same way as in other hematopoietic disorders.

Summary

Although no karyotypic abnormality is specific for PMF, certain chromosomes are involved preferentially in numerical or structural rearrangements. Some of these rearrangements have also been found in other hematologic disorders. On the other hand, the specific changes associated with acute myeloid leukemia of defined cell type have not been identified in any patients with PMF.

From the data available for analysis, the best prognosis in PMF was not associated with the presence of a normal karyotype at diagnosis. Patients with certain karyotypic changes had a better prognosis and others a worse prognosis than those with a normal karyotype.

More reports of cytogenetic studies in patients with MF are needed, despite the technical difficulties connected with this disorder, since the relatively few studies reported so far appear to provide useful information for the assessment of prognosis.

ACKNOWLEDGMENTS

We are grateful to Dr. B. R. Reeves for a constructive criticism of this review and to the departments of Medical Art and Photography at the Royal Marsden Hospital for preparation of the illustrations.

REFERENCES

1. Nowell, P. C., and Hungerford, D. A. (1960). A minute chromosome in human chronic granulocytic leukemia. *Science 132*: 1497.
2. Rowley, J. D. (1973). A new consistent chromosome abnormality in chronic myelogenous leukemia identified by quinacrine fluorescence and Giemsa staining. *Nature 243*: 290–293.
3. Lawler, S. D. (1982). Significance of chromosome abnormalities in leukemia. *Sem. Hematol. 19*: 257–272.
4. Fourth International Workshop on Chromosomes in Leukemia, 1982. (1984). Overview of association between chromosome pattern and cell morphology, age, sex and race. *Cancer Genet. Cytogenet. 11*: 265–274.
5. Groffen, J., Heisterkamp, N., Stephenson, J. R., van Kessel, A. G., de Klein, A., Grosveld, G., and Boostma, D. c-sis is translocated from chromosome 22 to chromosome 9 in chronic myelocytic leukemia. *J. Exp. Med. 158*: 9–15.
6. de Klein, A., van Kessel, A. G., Grosveld, G., Bartram, C. R., Hagemeijer, A., Bootsma, D., Spurr, N. K., Heisterkamp, N., Groffen, J., and Stephenson, J. R. (1982). A cellular oncogene is translocated to the Philadelphia chromosome in chronic myelocytic leukaemia. *Nature 300*: 765–767.
7. Caspersson, T., Gahrton, G., Lindsten, J., and Zech, L. (1970). Identification of the Philadelphia chromosome as a number 22 by quinacrine mustard fluorescence analysis. *Exp. Cell Res. 63*: 238–240.
8. Georgii, A., Thiele, J., and Vykoupil, K. F. (1980). Osteomyelofibrosis/-

sclerosis: A histological and cytogenetic study on core biopsies of the bone marrow. *Virchows Arch. A. Path. Anat. Histol. 389*: 269–286.

9. Cehreli, C., Ezdinli, E. Z., Li, C. Y., and Krmpotic, E. (1976). Blastic phase of agnogenic myeloid metaplasia simulating malignant lymphoma. *Cancer 38*: 1297–1305.
10. Brandt, L., Mitelman, F., and Panani, A. (1975). Cytogenetic differences between bone marrow and spleen in a case of agnogenic myeloid metaplasia developing blast crisis. *Scand. J. Haematol. 15*: 187–191.
10a. Mitelman, F., Brandt, L., and Nilsson, P. G. (1974). Cytogenetic evidence for splenic origin of blastic transformation in chronic myeloid leukemia. *Scand. J. Haematol. 13*: 89–92.
11. ISCN. (1978). An international system for human cytogenetic nomenclature. Birth defects: original article series, vol. XIV, no. 8. New York, The National Foundation.
12. Sandberg, A. A. (1980). *The Chromosomes in Human Cancer and Leukemia.* New York, Elsevier, pp. 354–362.
13. Nowell, P., Jensen, J., Gardner, F., Murphy, S., Chaganti, R. S. K., and German, J. (1976). Chromosome studies in "preleukemia". III. Myelofibrosis. *Cancer 38*: 1873–1881.
14. Besa, E. C., Nowell, P. C., Geller, N. L., and Gardner, F. H. (1982). Analysis of the androgen response of 23 patients with agnogenic myeloid metaplasia. *Cancer 49*: 308–313.
15. Whang-Peng, J., Lee, E., Knutsen, T., Chang, P., and Nienhuis, A. (1978). Cytogenetic studies in patients with myelofibrosis and myeloid metaplasia. *Leuk. Res. 2*: 41–56.
16. Rowley, J. D. (1977). Mapping of human chromosomal regions related to neoplasia: evidence from chromosomes 1 and 17. *Proc. Natl. Acad. Sci. USA 74*: 5729–5733.
17. Hsu, L. Y. F., Pinchiaroli, D., Gilbert, H. S., Wittman, R., and Hirschhorn, K. (1977). Partial trisomy of the long arm of chromosome 1 in myelofibrosis and polycythemia vera. *Am. J. Hematol. 2*: 375–383.
18. van den Berghe, H., Cassiman, H., David, G., Fryns, J. P., Michaux, J. L., and Sokal, G. (1974). Distinct haematological disorder with deletion of long arm of No. 5 chromosome. *Nature 251*: 437–438.
19. Rowley, J. D. (1976). 5q– acute myelogenous leukemia: Reply. *Blood 48*: 626.
20. Sieff, C. A., Chessells, J. M., Harvey, B. A. M., Pickthall, V. J., and Lawler, S. D. (1981). Monosomy 7 in childhood: A myeloproliferative disorder. *Br. J. Haematol. 49*: 235–249.
21. Rowley, J. D. (1973). Identification of a translocation with quinacrine fluorescence in a patient with acute leukemia. *Ann. Genet. 16*: 109–112.
22. Zech, L., Haglund, U., Nilsson, K., and Klein, G. (1976). Characteristic chromosomal abnormalities in biopsies and lymphoid cell lines from patients with Burkitt & non-Burkitt lymphomas. *Int. J. Cancer 17*: 47–56.

23. Berrebi, A., Dvilanski, A., and Chemke, J. (1983). Cytogenetic studies in Megakaryoblastic leukaemia. *Acta Haemat. 69*: 66–67.
24. Berger, R., Bernheim, A., Weh, H. J., Daniel, M. T., and Flandrin, G. (1979). Leucémie aiguë monocytaire avec anomalie du chromosome 11. *Nouv. Presse Med. 8*: 2836.
25. Engel, W., Merker, H., Schneider, G., and Wolf, U. (1968). Clonal occurrence of a chromosome Dq− in myelosclerosis with myeloid metaplasia. *Humangenetik 6*: 335–337.
26. Kohno, S. I., van den Berghe, H., and Sandberg, A. A. (1979). Chromosomes and causation of human cancer and leukemia. XXXI. Dq− deletions and their significance in proliferative disorders. *Cancer 43*: 1350–1357.
27. Borgström, G. H., Knuutila, S., Teerenhovi, L., and Vuopio, P. (1982). Interstitial deletion of chromosome 13 in myelofibrosis. Budapest, 19th Congress of International Society of Haematology, p. 268.
28. Reeves, B. R., Lobb, D. S., and Lawler, S. D. (1972). Identity of the abnormal F-group chromosome associated with polycythaemia vera. *Humangenetik 14*: 159–161.
29. Testa, J. R., Kinnealey, A., Rowley, J. D., Golde, D. W., and Potter, D. (1978). Deletion of the long arm of chromosome 20 [del(20)(q11)] in myeloid disorders. *Blood 52*: 868–877.
30. Third International Workshop on Chromosomes in Leukemia (1981). *Cancer Genet. Cytogenet. 4*: 95–142.
31. Sandberg, A. A. (1980). *The Chromosomes in Human Cancer and Leukaemia.* New York, Elsevier, pp. 267–275.
32. Carbonell, F., Ganser, A., and Heimpel, H. (1983). Cytogenetic studies in chronic myeloproliferative disorders. *Acta. Haematol. 69*: 145–151.
33. Lawler, S. D. (1980). Cytogenetic studies in Philadelphia chromosome-negative myeloproliferative disorders, particularly polycythaemia rubra vera. *Clin. Haematol. 9*: 159–173.
34. Hoppin, E. C., and Lewis, J. P. (1975). Polycythaemia rubra vera progressing to Ph1-positive chronic myelogenous leukemia. *Ann. Int. Med. 83*: 820–823.
35. Clough, V., Geary, C. G., Hashmi, K., Davson, J., and Knowlson, T. (1979). Myelofibrosis in chronic granulocytic leukaemia. *Br. J. Haematol. 42*: 515–526.
36. Sandberg, A. A. (1980). *The Chromosomes in Human Cancer and Leukemia.* New York, Elsevier, p. 207.
37. Holden, J. D., Garcia, U. G., Samuels, M., Dupin, C., Stallworth, B., and Anderson, E. (1971). Myelofibrosis with C monosomy of marrow elements in a child. *Am. J. Clin. Pathol. 55*: 573–579.
38. Evans, D. I. K. (1975). Acute myelofibrosis in children with Down's syndrome. *Arch. Dis. Childhood 50*: 458–462.
39. Hillman, F., and Forrester, R. M. (1968). Myelofibrosis simulating acute

leukaemia in a female infant with Down's syndrome. *Irish J. Med. Sci. 1* (7th Series): 167–173.

40. Ueda, K., Kawaguchi, Y., Kodama, M., Tanaka, Y., Usui, T., and Kamada, N. (1981). Primary myelofibrosis with myeloid metaplasia and cytogenetically abnormal clones in 2 children with Down's Syndrome. *Scand. J. Haematol. 27*: 152–158.
41. Nielsen, J. (1975). Chromosome examination of newborn children. Purpose and ethical aspects. *Humangenetik 26*: 215–222.
42. Pakkala, A., Ruutu, T., Partanen, S., Kovanen, R., Borgström, G. H., and Knuutila, S. (1983). Peripheral blood cells in the study of chromosome aberrations of patients with chronic myeloid leukaemia or myelofibrosis. *Acta. Haematol. 70*: 264–268.
43. Page, B. M., Watt, J. L., Reid, I. N., Davidson, R. J. L., and Walker, W. (1979). Clonal evolution of marker chromosomes in a case of myelofibrosis with myeloid metaplasia and myeloblastic transformation. *Acta Haematol. 61*: 301–309.
44. Ward, H. P., and Block, M. H. (1971). The natural history of agnogenic myeloid metaplasia (AMM) and a critical evaluation of its relationship with the myeloproliferative syndrome. *Medicine 50*: 357–420.
45. Clare, N., Elson, D., and Manhoff, L. (1982). Cytogenetic studies of peripheral myeloblasts and bone marrow fibroblasts in acute myelofibrosis. *Am. J. Clin. Pathol. 77*: 762–766.
46. Jacobson, R. J., Salo, A., and Fialkow, P. J. (1978). Agnogenic myeloid metaplasia: A clonal proliferation of hematopoietic stem cells with secondary myelofibrosis. *Blood 51*: 189–194.
47. Nowell, P. C., and Finan, J. B. Cytogenetics of acute and chronic myelofibrosis. *Virchows Arch. B. Cell Pathol. 29*: 45–50.
48. Ruutu, T., Partanen, S., and Knuutila, S. (1983). Clonal karyotype abnormalities in erythroid and granulocyte-monocyte precursors in polycythaemia vera and myelofibrosis. *Scand. J. Haematol. 31*: 253–256.
49. van Dyke, D. L., Abraham, J. P., Maeda, K., Weiss, L., and Poel, M. (1981). Multiple active X chromosomes in myelofibrosis with myeloid metaplasia. *Cancer Genet. Cytogenet. 3*: 137–144.
50. Ganser, A., and Carbonell, F. (1982). Cytogenetic studies using HPCM-stimulated short-term liquid cultures of circulating hemopoietic precursor cells in patients with myelofibrosis. *Blut 44*: 111–114.
51. Bird, T., and Proctor, S. J. (1976). Malignant myelosclerosis: myeloproliferative disorder or leukemia? *Am. J. Clin. Pathol. 67*: 516–520.
52. Nowell, P., and Finan, J. (1978). Chromosome studies in preleukemic states. IV. Myeloproliferative versus cytopenic disorders. *Cancer 42*: 2254–2261.
53. Peto, R., Pike, M. C., Armitage, P., Breslow, N. E., Cox, D., Howard, S. V., Mantel, N., McPherson, K., Peto, J., and Smith, P. G. (1977). De-

sign and analysis of randomized clinical trials requiring prolonged observation of each patient. *Br. J. Cancer 35*: 1–39.
54. Rowley, J. D., Golomb, H. M., and Vardiman, J. W. (1981). Nonrandom chromosome abnormalities in acute leukemia and dysmyelopoietic syndromes in patients with previously treated malignant disease. *Blood 58*: 759–767.
55. Hagemeijer, A., Hahlen, K., Smit, E. M. E., and van Zanen, G. E. (1980). C-Group chromosome abnormalities in bone marrow cells of three children with dyshaematopoiesis of unknown origin. *Br. J. Haematol. 46*: 377–385.
56. Davidson, W. M., and Knight, L. A. (1973). Acquired trisomy 9. *Lancet i*: 1510.
57. Findley, L., Kurnick, J. E., Peakman, D. C., and Robinson, A. (1979). Chromosome deletion [46,XX,del(20)(q11)] in agnogenic myeloid metaplasia. *Hum. Genet. 47*: 207–211.
58. Fleischman, E. W., Prigogina, E. L., Volkova, M. A., and Kulagina, O. E. (1979). Chromosomal marker 20q– in cases of osteomyelosclerosis and CML. *Hum. Genet. 50*: 101–104.
59. Hsu, L. Y. F., Greenberg, M. L., Kohan, S., and Wittman, R. (1979). Trisomy 13 in bone marrow cells in acute myelocytic leukemia and myelofibrosis. *Clin. Genet. 15*: 327–331.
60. Gahrton, G., Friberg, K., Lindsten, J., and Zech, L. (1978). Duplication of part of the long arm of chromosome 1 in myelofibrosis terminating in acute myeloblastic leukemia. *Hereditas 88*: 1–5.
61. Geraedts, J. P. M., den Ottolander, G. J., Ploem, J. E., and Muntinghe, O. G. (1980). An identical translocation between chromosome 1 and 7 in three patients with myelofibrosis and myeloid metaplasia. *Br. J. Haematol. 44*: 569–575.
62. de Greef, I., Geraedts, J. P. M., and Leeksma, C. H. W. (1982). Malignant hematologic disorders in two Robertsonian 13;14 translocation carriers. *Cancer Genet. Cytogenet. 7*: 181–184.
63. Miyamoto, K., Hamasaki, K., Kitajima, K., Adachi, T., Tanaka, T., and Santo, J. (1981). Abnormalities of chromosome no. 1 related to blood dyscrasias: study of 10 cases. *Acta Med. Okayama 35*: 137–141.
64. Moake, J. L., Lebos, H., and Warren, R. J. (1974). Chromosomal abnormalities in a patient with adolescent myelofibrosis. *Acta Haematol. 52*: 173–179.
65. Rosenthal, D. S., and Moloney, W. C. (1977). Occurrence of acute leukaemia in myeloproliferative disorders. *Br. J. Haematol. 36*: 373–382.
66. Whaun, J. M., Lin, C. C., Biederman, B., Cornish, S. J., and Dundas, J. B. (1981). Myeloproliferative disorder with unusual marrow chromosome constitution. *Cancer 48*: 1164–1169.
67. Aide, Y., Shumao, L., Ju, Y., Hongbao, F., Bianming, W., Jun, G.,

Shaoyu, Z. (1981). Significance of chromosome studies in leukemia: karyotype analysis of 28 cases of leukemia and 2 cases of myelofibrosis. *Acta Acad. Med. Wuhan 1*: 7–15.

68. Baravika, I., Bondare, D., and Jaworkowsky, L. (1980). Die Trisomie des langen Armes ersten Chromosoms bei einem Patienten mit primärer Myelofibrose wahrend der Blastenkrise. *Folia Haematol. Leipzig 107*: 885–889.
69. Schmid, E., and Kohler, J. (1984). Involvement of chromosomes 1 and 11 in three cases with myeloproliferative diseases. *Cancer Genet. Cytogenet. 11*: 121–123.
70. Sessarego, M., Ajmar, F., Ravazzolo, R., Bianchi Scarra, G. L., Garre, C., and Boccaccio, P. (1983). Coincidence between fragile site expression and interstitial deletion of chromosome 11 in a case of myelofibrosis. *Hum. Genet. 63*: 299-301.
71. Bartoli, E., Massarelli, G., Soggia, G., Tanda, F., and Vianello, M. G. (1979). Acute agnogenic myeloid metaplasia with chromosomal abnormalities. *Acta. Haematol. 62*: 206–213.
72. den Ottolander, G. J., te Velde, J., Brederoo, P., Geraedts, J. P. M., Slee, P. H. T., Willemze, R., Zwaan, F. E., Haak, H. L., Muller, H. P., and Bieger, R. (1979). Megakaryoblastic leukaemia (acute myelofibrosis): a report of three cases. *Br. J. Haematol. 42*: 9–20.
73. Shah, I., Mayeda, K., Koppitch, F., Mahmood, S., and Nemitz, B. (1982). Karyotypic polymorphism in acute myelofibrosis. *Blood 60*: 841–844.
74. Najfeld, V., Price, T. H., Adamson, J. W., and Fialkow, P. J. (1978). Myelofibrosis with complex chromosome abnormality in a patient with erythrocytosis due to hemoglobin Rainier treated with ^{32}P. *Am. J. Haematol. 5*: 63–69.
75. Rowley, J. D. (1975). Abnormalities of chromosome 1 in myeloproliferative disorders. *Cancer 36*: 1748–1757.
76. Mecucci, C., Vermaelen, K., Tricot, G., Louwagie, A., Michaux, J. L., Bosly, A., Thomas, J., Barbieri, D., and van den Berghe, H. (1983). 3q−, 3q+ anomaly in malignant proliferations in humans. *Cancer Genet. Cytogenet. 9*: 367–381.

10

Treatment of Myelofibrosis

MURRAY N. SILVERSTEIN, M.D.
Mayo Medical School, Rochester, Minnesota

INTRODUCTION

In 1984, myelofibrosis is still an incurable disease: treatment is based primarily upon the symptoms the patient displays. Approximately 30% of patients will be asymptomatic at diagnosis (1). These patients require careful observation; as a rule no therapy has been prescribed at this stage.

Sooner or later the majority of patients with myelofibrosis manifest symptoms associated with anemia, pressure from the enlarged spleen, bleeding, portal hypertension, ascites, bone pain, or hypermetabolism. Successful management of each of these problems depends upon appropriate evaluation of the underlying symptoms.

THE ANEMIC PATIENT

It has been estimated that 60% of patients with myelofibrosis will become anemic during their clinical course (1). For 95% of the time, this anemia will be normocytic and normochromic while 5% of patients may manifest iron deficiency anemia. The British literature (2) has quoted a significant occurrence of macrocytic anemia secondary to folic acid deficiency. In the United States, however, macrocytic anemia has been a very rare occurrence in patients with myelofibrosis.

Before embarking on any therapy in an anemic patient with myelofibrosis, it is mandatory to determine the total blood volume with red cell mass and plasma volume. As with other splenomegalic states, the increasing size of the spleen may be accompanied by a marked expansion in plasma volume. Blood volume determinations may thus demonstrate anemia to be purely on a "dilutional" basis. Such patients with "dilutional anemia" require no treatment of the apparent anemia per se.

Patients who have low red cell masses with normocytic normochromic anemia should be considered for treatment. Approximately 95% of such patients will have ineffective erythropoiesis (1, 3). Additionally, 50% will have shortened red cell survival. In those patients with ineffective erythropoiesis, androgen therapy is indicated. Currently, oral androgens are initiated in patients with or without thrombocytopenia. Of the available oral androgens, Oxymetholone in doses of 50 mg four times a day, or fluoxymesterone in doses of 10 mg three times a day may be beneficial. In patients without thrombocytopenia, it is worthwhile considering intramuscular testosterone enanthate which may be effective in doses of 400 mg intramuscularly every 3-4 weeks. Responses to androgen therapy may be delayed for up to 3-4 months; therefore, one should continue these agents for at least this period of time. Careful monitoring of liver function tests, especially serum glutamic oxalacetic transaminase and alkaline phosphatase is necessary during androgen therapy.

In patients with shortened red cell survival, adrenal steroids are helpful. We have used doses of 10 mg of prednisone three times a day for such patients. One must keep in mind that one-half of the patients with normocytic, normochromic anemia complicating myelofibrosis will have a bipronged mechanism for this anemia, i.e., ineffective erythropoiesis plus shortened red cell survival. Thus, these patients will require a combination of androgen therapy with adrenal steroids. Occasionally, patients with myelofibrosis may develop severe hemolytic anemia refractory to steroid therapy. Such patients are candidates for splenectomy. Five of nine patients so treated in our group had a successful rise of hemoglobin following the procedure (4).

In patients with iron deficiency anemia, the underlying etiology of the iron deficiency must be identified. In myelofibrosis, peptic ulceration or esophageal varices may be the etiology for iron deficiency and these lesions must be treated. Occasionally, work-up of a patient with iron deficiency anemia and myelofibrosis may uncover evidence of an occult gastrointestinal carcinoma requiring surgery. After correcting the underlying cause of anemia, oral iron therapy is indicated. My preference in oral iron therapy has been ferrous sulfate, 300 mg per day for at least 3 months.

In those rare patients with macrocytic anemia, the underlying etiology must be determined. If folic acid or B_{12} deficiency are discovered, replacement therapy with these vitamins is required.

THE PATIENT WITH MECHANICAL SPLENOMEGALY

Approximately 23% of patients with myelofibrosis will develop a progressively enlarging painful spleen (1). These patients may complain of severe progressive pain, especially when the spleen enlarges to fill the entire left side of the abdomen. Many patients will develop serious digestive disturbances, especially early satiety with easy filling and subsequent weight loss. Some patients may present with acute severe pain secondary to splenic infarction. Rarely, patients may develop intractable diarrhea as the result of the enlarged spleen pressing on the left colon.

In patients with progressive mechanical splenomegaly and inexorable pain, methods to shrink the spleen have been utilized. In the past these have included chemotherapy in the form of busulfan (5) and, more recently, hydroxyurea (6). Approximately two-thirds of patients treated will have a shrinking of the spleen, but with discontinuation of these agents, rapid enlargement of the spleen will recur.

Radiation therapy should also be considered in patients with profound mechanical splenomegaly (7). In patients with acute splenic infarction who do not respond to simple analgesia, focal radiation therapy over the spleen in doses of 25-50 rads daily for 4-5 days may produce gratifying results (8). Additionally, those patients with a huge painful spleen in whom splenectomy cannot be considered may be benefited by a cautious trial of radiotherapy (8).

Our experience suggests that patients with mechanical splenomegaly with profoundly enlarged spleens are best treated by splenectomy (4). Whenever splenectomy is contemplated an all-encompassing work-up is required. The patients must be considered acceptable in terms of cardiac, hepatic, renal, and metabolic risks. All patients must have an extensive coagulation survey; this must include assays for Factors V, VIII, fibrin-split products, and platelet function. All patients with myelofibrosis will demonstrate qualitative platelet abnormalities (9). These patients are nonetheless candidates for splenectomy but they may require to be covered by an adrenal steroid preparation preoperatively and platelet transfusions at the time of surgery after the splenic pedicle has been clamped. In patients with "inapparent DIC," surgery is contraindicated (4). The operation itself must be considered as a major procedure, so that only a senior staff person who has done this type of surgery many times in the past should perform the operation. As our group has reported, 27 of 28 patients who had splenectomy for mechanical splenomegaly have had an excellent response from this procedure (4).

THE BLEEDING PATIENT

Clinically, serious bleeding may complicate myelofibrosis in approximately 16% of patients. This may be multifactorial. Invariably patients with myelofibrosis will have qualitative platelet dysfunction secondary to aggregation abnormalities (1). In addition, thrombocytopenia may develop in upwards of 35% of patients, and inapparent DIC, as mentioned above, occurs in 12% of patients. In those patients with qualitative functional abnormalities, the use of platelet transfusions and adrenal steroids is indicated for serious bleeding or in preparing a patient for impending surgery. Patients with thrombocytopenia secondary to either or both marrow failure and hypersplenism will often be managed with adrenal steroids. In patients with life-threatening thrombocytopenia who do not respond to steroids, splenectomy may be helpful (4). No general rule can be laid down for managing patients with myelofibrosis and DIC. Patients with inapparent DIC require no treatment, but surgery is totally contraindicated. In patients who develop DIC secondary to infection or other etiologies, treatment is best conducted by controlling the underlying etiology and using replacement therapy with platelets and Factors V and VIII.

THE PATIENT WITH PORTAL HYPERTENSION

Portal hypertension may complicate myelofibrosis in 6–8% of patients (10). With the development of this potentially catastrophic problem, careful assessment of the patient is mandatory. The mechanism of portal hypertension in myelofibrosis may be two-fold: (a) secondary to massive increased blood flow from the spleen to the liver, i.e., forward flow, portal hypertension, or (b) secondary to intrahepatic block as a result of postnecrotic cirrhosis, which may follow transfusional hepatitis. Clinically, portal hypertension is characterized by either the presence of esophageal varices or ascites, or both.

The treatment of portal hypertension in myelofibrosis is surgical. Our experience (10) suggests that this complication is secondary to forward flow in 70% of patients, and in 30% of patients it is the result of intrahepatic block. When at surgery forward-flow portal hypertension is demonstrable by marked increase in hepatic blood flow and the collapse of varices following clamping of the splenic vessels, the simple expedient of splenectomy will lead to beneficial effects (10). If the portal hypertension is secondary to intrahepatic block, our group has favored splenorenal shunt as the decompression procedure of choice. Our data have shown limited survival in patients treated medically with variceal bleeding, but prolonged survival in patients treated surgically (10).

THE PATIENT WITH ASCITES, BONE PAIN, OR HYPERMETABOLISM

Ascites may complicate myelofibrosis in 6–8% of patients. The mechanism of ascites may be two-fold, and the underlying etiology of the ascites must be determined so that effective therapy can be provided. In some patients, ascites will be secondary to portal hypertension, and management of these patients should be directed to the portal hypertension. In all patients with myelofibrosis, a peritoneal tap and careful study of the ascitic fluid is mandatory. If one finds megakaryocytes in spun samples of ascitic fluid, the mechanism of ascites is the result of peritoneal implants of myeloid metaplasia (11). Treatment of peritoneal implants of myeloid metaplasia consists of abdominal radiation. We have found that treating these patients with fractional doses of radiation at the level of 25 rad per day rotating into four quadrants of the abdomen is extremely effective. Continuous therapy with a total dose of up to 500–1000 rad may also be very rewarding.

When patients with myelofibrosis develop bone pain, one must be extremely guarded as to prognosis. Our experience suggests that this complication represents leukemic transformation in evolution (1). In these patients with severe bone pain, biopsies at painful sites may reveal cultures of pure leukemic blasts. The mechanism of pain appears to be a result of periosteal invasion by blast cells. Recommended treatment for bone pain is by focal radiation therapy in doses of 25–50 rad per day for several days. This often results in gratifying relief.

Hypermetabolism is not an unusual phenomenon in myelofibrosis. Symptoms of asthenia, weight loss, and sweating may occur. Such patients may benefit from the use of low-dose adrenal steroids, e.g., 10–20 mg of prednisone a day and/or the use of low doses of hydroxyurea, i.e., 500–1000 mg/day. The latter agent may be effective in reducing spleen size and decreasing metabolic activity in hematopoietic sties.

NEW APPROACHES TO THERAPY

Rapid strides have been made in the understanding of the biosynthesis of collagen in this disorder. Biochemically, as myelofibrosis progresses, there is a parallel insolubilization of collagen leading to progressive fibrosis (12). Conversion of soluble to insoluble collagen requires the monoamine oxidase of lysine to produce lysyl aldehydes from lysine. Lysyl aldehydes then cross-link collagen, resulting in the formation of insoluble collagen.

Monoamine oxidase inhibitors prevent the formation of lysyl aldehydes. Examples of such compounds include penicillamine and beta-amino propionitrile (BAPN). Chelation of lysyl aldehydes can be accomplished by penicillamine and BAPN. The interference to lysyl aldehyde formation and subsequent cross-linkage of collagen may be expected to decrease fibrous tissue deposition and in fact this occurs. Dickson et al. (13) have employed D-penicillamine in a prospective double-blind randomized trial in patients with primary biliary cirrhosis in which 115 patients were randomized to placebo and 113 patients were randomized to D-penicillamine. Significant improvement in survival after 2 years of therapy has been observed in the D-penicillamine-treated group. Additionally, patients treated with D-penicillamine have shown significant decreases in serum glutamic oxyloacetic transaminase, alkaline phosphatase, gamma globulin, and erythrocyte sedimentation rate. BAPN has been observed to decrease esophageal strictures resulting from lye burns.

Colchicine, by its ability to disrupt microtubules, produces a decreased rate of secretion of procollagen (14). Additionally, this agent increases the secretion of collagenases by cultures of rheumatoid synovium. By both of these functions, colchicine may indeed produce an antifibrosing effect. Recently, Rojkind (14) reported significant improvements in patients with scleroderma treated with colchicine.

Since there is no specific treatment available for myelofibrosis, and since the disorder is characterized by progressive marrow fibrosis, it would seem realistic to consider using antifibrosing agents in this syndrome in an attempt to reverse the fibrotic process in the bone marrow. Newer techniques have been recently developed to quantify bone marrow fibrosis (12). In addition, new immunohistochemical techniques are available to determine the type of collagen produced in the marrow of patients with myelofibrosis (15). Finally, a procollagen fragment in the blood has been thought to mirror the activity of fibroblasts in the marrow (16). At the present time, trials of penicillamine and colchicine are underway at our institution. The initial group of patients being treated are those who are essentially asymptomatic. At the present time, the trials are too early in evolution to determine the effectiveness of this approach. It is planned that patients will be treated at least 1–2 years with penicillamine or colchicine.

Summary

The management of patients with myelofibrosis is complex. It is extremely important for the clinician to determine the underlying mechanism producing a patient's symptoms. Anemic patients with myelofibrosis who demonstrate ineffective erythropoiesis may respond to androgen therapy. In patients with a hemolytic component to their anemia, adrenal steroids are helpful. Patients with mechanical splenomegaly are probably best treated by splenectomy. In those patients who are not candidates for splenectomy, consideration of chemotherapy and radiotherapy are indicated. Patients with acute splenic infarction are best managed with radiotherapy.

The underlying cause of bleeding must be determined in patients with myelofibrosis before therapy is undertaken. In patients who bleed because of platelet functional abnormalities, the use of adrenal steroids and platelet transfusions is helpful. Thrombocytopenic patients refractory to adrenal steroids may respond to splenectomy. Patients with inapparent DIC are not candidates for surgery.

Before treating a patient with portal hypertension, the underlying mechanism must be determined. If the patient has forward-flow portal hypertension, splenectomy will produce gratifying results. In patients with intrahepatic block, a systemic decompressive shunt procedure is indicated and splenorenal shunts are worthwhile. Patients may develop ascites secondary to portal hypertension or to peritoneal implants of myeloid metaplasia. In those patients with intractable ascites and portal hypertension, surgical decompression is indicated. In patients with peritoneal implants of myeloid metaplasia, radiotherapy is the treatment of choice.

Patients who develop severe bone pain with myeloid metaplasia tend to be entering a leukemic transformation. Biopsies at painful sites often will demonstrate cultures of leukemic blasts. Focal radiation for the control of pain in these patients may be extremely helpful. Hypermetabolism is a common concomitant of myelofibrosis. The use of small doses of adrenal steroids and/or hydroxyurea may be worthwhile for this problem.

At the current time, a new approach to the treatment of myelofibrosis is underway at our institution. Patients are being treated with the antifibrosing agents penicillamine or colchicine. Data on this new approach should be forthcoming within the next 1-2 years.

REFERENCES

1. Silverstein, M. N. (1975). *Agnogenic Myeloid Metaplasia*, Acton, Massachusetts, Publishing Science Group, Inc., 126 pp.
2. Hoffbrand, A. V., Chanarin, I., Kremenchuzky, S., et al. (1968). Megaloblastic anemia in myelosclerosis. *Q. J. Med. 37*: 493–516.
3. Najean, Y., Caccione, R., Castro-Malaspina, H., et al. (1978). Erythrokinetic studies in myelofibrosis. *Br. J. Haematol. 40*: 205–217.

4. Silverstein, M. N., and ReMine, W. H. (1979). Splenectomy in myeloid metaplasia. *Blood 55*: 515–518.
5. Ward, H. P., and Block, M. H. (1979). The natural history of agnogenic myeloid metaplasia (AMM) and a critical evaluation of its relationship with the myeloproliferative syndrome. *Medicine 50*: 357–420.
6. Laszlo, J., et al. (1983). The use of hydroxyurea in myelofibrosis. Minutes of Polycythemia Vera Study Group, November, 1983.
7. Silverstein, M. N. (1983). Agnogenic Myeloid Metaplasia. In *Hematology*, third edition. Edited by W. J. Williams. New York, McGraw-Hill, pp. 214–218.
8. Silverstein, M. N. (1977). Control of hypersplenism and painful splenomegaly in myeloid metaplasia by irradiation. *Int. J. Radiat. Onc. Biol. Phys. 2*: 1221–1222.
9. Didisheim, P., and Bunting, D. (1966). Abnormal platelet function in myelofibrosis. *Am. J. Clin. Path. 45*: 566–573.
10. Silverstein, M. N. (1981). Portal hypertension (PH) in agnogenic myeloid metaplasia (AMM). *Blood 58*(152a): #520, December.
11. Gorshein, D., and Brauer, M. J. (1969). Ascites in myeloid metaplasia due to ectopic peritoneal implantation. *Cancer 23*: 1408–1412.
12. Charron, D., Palent, L., Couty, M. C., et al. (1979). Biochemical and histological analysis of bone marrow collagen in myelofibrosis. *Br. J. Haematol. 41*: 151–161.
13. Dickson, E. R., Baldus, W. P., and Wiesner, R. H. Primary biliary cirrhosis, D-Penicillamine Trial and Pharmacokinetics Renewal Grant, 5 R01, AM 19448–07.
14. Rojkind, M. (1985). Anti-inflammatory and antifibrogenic actions of Colchicine. Myelofibrosis and the Biology of the Connective Tissue. A symposium. November 11–12, 1982, New York (in press).
15. Gay, S., Gay, R. E., and Prchal, J. T. (1985). Immunohistochemical studies of bone marrow collagen. Myelofibrosis and the Biology of the Connective Tissue. A Symposium. November 11–12, 1982, New York (in press).
16. Hochweiss, S., Fruchtman, S., Hahn, E. G., et al. (1983). Increased serum procollagen III aminoterminal peptide in myelofibrosis. *Am. J. Haematol. 15*: 343–351.

Index